Health *and* Health Care Inequities

A Critical Political Economy Perspective

Health *and* Health Care Inequities

A Critical Political Economy Perspective

Arnel M. Borras

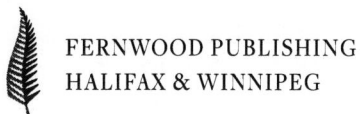
FERNWOOD PUBLISHING
HALIFAX & WINNIPEG

Copyright © 2025 Arnel M. Borras

All rights reserved. No part of this book may be reproduced or transmitted in any form by any means without permission in writing from the publisher, except by a reviewer, who may quote brief passages in a review.

Copyediting: Brenda Conroy
Cover Design: John van der Woude
Text Design: Lauren Jeanneau
Printed and bound in the UK

Published in North America by Fernwood Publishing
2970 Oxford Street, Halifax, Nova Scotia, B3L 2W4
Halifax and Winnipeg
www.fernwoodpublishing.ca

Fernwood Publishing Company Limited gratefully acknowledges the financial support of the Government of Canada through the Canada Book Fund and the Canada Council for the Arts. We acknowledge the Province of Manitoba for support through the Manitoba Publishers Marketing Assistance Program and the Book Publishing Tax Credit. We acknowledge the Nova Scotia Department of Communities, Culture and Heritage for support through the Publishers Assistance Fund.

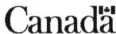 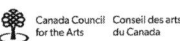 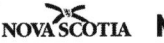 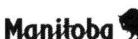

Library and Archives Canada Cataloguing in Publication

Title: Health and health care inequities : a critical political economy perspective / Arnel M. Borras.
Names: Borras, Arnel M., author.
Description: Includes bibliographical references and index.
Identifiers: Canadiana (print) 20240483413 | Canadiana (ebook) 20240483421 | ISBN 9781773637266 (softcover) | ISBN 9781773637280 (PDF)
Subjects: LCSH: Public health—Social aspects. | LCSH: Equality—Health aspects. | LCSH: Health services accessibility. | LCSH: Social medicine. | LCSH: Medical policy. | LCSH: Social justice.
Classification: LCC RA418 .B67 2025 | DDC 362.1—dc23

To you, the reader —
my fellow traveller on this journey of discovery and growth.
Together, let us ascend towards new heights. Onwards and upwards!

Contents

Acknowledgements viii

Introduction 1

1 | Social Determinants of Health Inequities 4
    The Social Determinants of Health 4
    The State of Health Inequities 7
    Notes 16

2 | Neoliberalism and Canada's Housing Policies 18
    Neoliberalism 20
    Historicizing Canada's Housing Policies 22
    The Impact of Neoliberal Housing Policies 25
    Neoliberalism and the State of Housing Insecurity 27
    Further Reflection 30
    Notes 32

3 | Neoliberalism and Canada's Health Care System 34
    Transition from Private to Public Health Care System 34
    Tug of War toward Socialist-Oriented Publicly Funded
    Universal Health Care 35
    The Continuing Private War against Universal Health Care 36
    Toward Privatized Health Care or Socialized Medicine? 39
    The Canada Health Act 41
    Health Care Policies in the Neoliberal Era 47
    Further Reflection 49
    Notes 50

4 | Political Power and Policy Advocacy 51
    Health Politics 51
    Political Participation and Representation 52
    Unequal Power and Politics 53
    Policy Change Approaches 55
    Unequal Resources, Unequal Policy Influence 59
    Further Reflection 65
    Note 66

5 | The Role of Evidence and Ideas 67
   Policy Paradigms and Policy Ideas 67
   Six Travelling Ideas 69
   Challenges with the Journeys of Ideas 71
   The Subordinate Role of Evidence and Research-Informed Ideas 73

6 | A Critical Political Economy Approach 82
   Capitalism and Its Impact on Health 83
   Capitalism–Imperialism–Colonialism–Racism Nexus 87
   Capitalism–Colonialism Nexus and Health Divide 90
   Capitalism–Racism Nexus and Health Divide 91
   Capitalism–Sexism Nexus and Health Divide 93
   The Intricate Web of Capitalism-Colonialism-Racism-Sexism 95
   Notes 98

7 | Searching for Socialism 100
   Welfare Systems in Capitalism 100
   Key Metrics across Welfare State Regimes 103
   Lessons from Welfare State Regimes and Neoliberalism 110
   Pathways to Addressing Health Inequities 113
   Circling and Countering Capitalism for Health Equity 117
   Further Reflection 119
   Note 120

8 | Mobilizing for Health Equity 121
   The Essence of Socialism 121
   Health Activism toward Socialism 123
   Our Minimum Demands 128
   Beyond Policy Change Limitations 130
   Conclusions 133

References 136
Index 154

Acknowledgements

This book represents not only the culmination of my efforts but also a rich tapestry woven from the generosity and wisdom of many. I am forever grateful to my doctoral dissertation research participants, who entrusted me with their stories and insights. My deepest thanks go to John Clarke, William Carroll, Trevor Hancock, Cathy Crowe, David Hulchanski, the late Leo Panitch, Pat Armstrong, Sam Gindin, Luin Goldring, Kwame McKenzie, Sheila Block, Akwatu Khenti, Sharleen Stewart, Greg Albo, Natalie Mehra, Michael Hurley, Jonah Gindin, Toba Bryant, and the anonymous interviewees. Your willingness to share your lived experiences has been the cornerstone of this endeavour.

My esteemed dissertation committee members, Dennis Raphael, Marina Morrow, and Jessica Vorstermans, have been unwavering sources of guidance and support. Your patience and wisdom have steered me through the twists and turns of my scholarly journey. Thank you to all my teachers and mentors inside and outside the academic world.

I am profoundly grateful to Errol Sharpe for his keen insights and thoughtful feedback, which have greatly enriched the book's depth and clarity. Thank you also to Sam Gindin and Herman Rosenfeld for their constructive comments, which have further strengthened the book. I thank my comrades at the Leo Panitch School for Socialist Education and the Socialist Project for welcoming me and enhancing my understanding and analysis through valuable discussions. Your support has been invaluable.

I am deeply grateful to the Fernwood Publishing team for their support during the production and marketing of my book. Special thanks to Art Bouman, Brenda Conroy, Debbie Mathers, Lauren Jeanneau, Anumeha Gokhale, Beverley Rach, and Errol Sharpe for their dedication and expertise. Your guidance was instrumental in bringing this project to life.

Lastly, to my cherished family, relatives, comrades, friends, co-workers, and classmates — your boundless support, encouragement, and belief in my vision have been the bedrock upon which this endeavour stands. Thank you for walking this path with me and breathing life into these pages.

Introduction

Health inequities — preventable differences in health among different social classes and groups — persist despite efforts to understand and address them. Attempts to narrow these health gaps through research and policies have not been successful. Poor working and living conditions contribute to higher rates of illness, disease, and death, which are significant public health concerns. Tackling these inequities is crucial to achieving better health for all.

This book discusses how social factors like class, race, gender, age, and where people live affect their health differently. It demonstrates that improving health for all requires looking beyond capitalist-focused policies. The book concentrates on Canada's health care system, often considered fair. Using a critical political economy approach, I examine how capitalist power, worker and community movements, and government decisions shape health policies. My arguments are supported by evidence from various sources, including existing literature and insights from in-depth interviews I performed with leading Canadian scholars and activists.

This study shows that the unequal distribution of societal wealth and resources, influenced by Big Capital and state policies, creates and maintains health inequities. The findings challenge the idea that research and evidence mainly drive policies affecting social and health issues such as housing, health care, and work conditions. Capitalism, infused with colonialism, racism, sexism, patriarchy, gender discrimination, and unfair resource allocation by governments, is the root cause of health inequities.

A stark contrast in life expectancy reveals the depth of health inequities. Japan has an average life span of 84 years, surpassing Canada's 82 years. Lesotho stands at a mere 51 years (WHO 2023, 51), lagging by over three decades compared to Canada. Class, race, gender, and other social locations shape health outcomes. For example, from 1996 to 2011, Canada's life expectancy gap between the richest and poorest widened by a year for men and two years for women (Bushnik, Tjepkema, and Martel 2020, 8). Residents of Nunavut live an average of ten fewer years than the national average (Statistics Canada 2018, 1). These figures challenge the notion of a uniformly prosperous Canadian health care system.

Chapter 1 deeply examines health inequities, going beyond mere description. It combines theoretical discussions with rich statistical data to show how social and economic inequalities impact health. It explores how differences in class, race, and gender create health inequities through the unequal distribution of the social determinants of health. The facts and figures clearly show that class is the primary driver of socioeconomic and health inequities, but race and gender, intertwined with class, exacerbate these inequities, particularly in the Canadian context.

Chapter 2 introduces three contending economic theories and practices, highlighting the emergence of neoliberalism. It historicizes Canada's housing policies from the early 1900s to the National Housing Strategy Act of 2019, demonstrating how housing insecurity and homelessness disproportionately harm certain groups' health. The chapter underscores the shift from Keynesian to neoliberal policy approaches, which led to housing support cuts and the end of federal housing programs, exacerbating housing problems for many. It advocates for socialized housing as a solution.

Chapter 3 examines Canada's transformation from a predominantly private to a publicly funded health care system. It discusses how the system initially had robust support from workers, communities, and governments but deteriorated over time, leading to a health care crisis. The chapter highlights the influence of Big Capital and the state in shaping policies that make health services more privatized, which is the main factor driving this crisis. It advocates for expanding public health care to prevent ongoing erosion of the health care system.

In Chapter 4, I combine existing literature and insights from my interviewees to investigate how different groups, such as businesses, community organizations, and governments, vie to shape policies that are to their benefit. Looking at the United States, United Kingdom, Australia, and Canada, the chapter shows that some groups have more wealth and power than others, leading to unfair health policies. It demonstrates that the rich and powerful have too much influence over state decisions, worsening health inequities.

Chapter 5 assesses how research and evidence influence policies on health inequities. The chapter discusses pioneering studies by Katherine Smith (2007, 2013a, 2013b, 2014) that examine how ideas are integrated into policies addressing health inequities. I include excerpts from my interviewees to add depth to the discussion and compare literature and interview data findings to provide perspectives that support and fill gaps in health research.

Chapter 6 shows that capitalism — integrally intertwined with racism and sexism — is the fundamental cause of health inequities. It criticizes capitalist state policies that help rich people get richer, exacerbating class, race, and gender inequalities. The chapter encourages workers' and people's movements to fight against these injustices, confronting capitalism, racism, and sexism altogether to help prevent and reduce health inequities.

In Chapter 7, I compare welfare state health care systems leaning towards socialism with those in Christian, democratic, liberal, and former fascist countries, showing how these systems affect socioeconomic inequalities and health. The aim is to determine if socialist ideas and policies can effectively address health inequities. Highlighting Erik Olin Wright's (2015, 2018) thoughts on modern movements against capitalism, which combine various types of struggles within and outside the government, the chapter posits that a socialist approach to health equity is achievable.

The last chapter focuses on health activism, urging health care workers to tackle health inequities. It argues that health activism promoting socialism will help meet urgent health needs and is an intelligent way to improve society. It suggests policy changes like improving working conditions, increasing social support, providing socialized housing, and expanding health services to reduce health inequities. Socialist principles influence these health-related public policy ideas.

The changes we want in policies are not capitalist; they are socialist. Even though these policies may seem like small steps within the current system, they are socialist practices and ideas. This approach serves two purposes: it makes immediate improvements under capitalism and paves the way for a socialist system that focuses on meeting people's needs, not making profits. The chapter supports a platform from the Socialist Project Labour Movement promoting solidarity among workers, making labour movements more democratic, and forming a socialist political party. To achieve health for all, we need to replace capitalism with socialism.

This book aims to spark thoughtful conversation and collaboration by moving away from capitalism to improve society and health. Health is not just about nursing and medicine; it is integrally connected to economic, political, cultural, and institutional systems. Moreover, it encompasses philosophy and ethics. Capitalism's focus on individualism and competition harms people and the environment, making it all but impossible to achieve health equity. We must work together to envision and create a new world that ensures fairer and better health for all.

CHAPTER ONE

Social Determinants of Health Inequities

What are health inequities? Where and when do they occur? Why do they happen? Let us explore these questions to work towards fairer health for everyone. Many researchers have investigated the reasons behind health inequities and proposed various prevention strategies. However, studies show that these inequities continue to exist worldwide despite efforts to solve them. Even though governments have tried to address the problem with public policies, health inequities remain. One helpful way to tackle these inequities is to examine the socioeconomic, political, and cultural factors affecting health.

The Social Determinants of Health

The social determinants of health encompass life's conditions from the uterus to death. The "toxic combination of poor social policies, unfair economics, and bad politics" affecting the social determinants of health results in unjust health inequalities (WHO 2008, 35). The unequal distribution of the social determinants of health, such as employment and working conditions, income and wealth, housing, food, education, social support, and health services contributes to health inequities (Raphael et al. 2020). Health inequities mainly result from unequal social relations of power shaping the distribution of the social determinants of health among social classes and groups.

Wages

A look at the average weekly earnings in 2015 of Canadian-born workers aged 25 to 44 reveals that, after adjusting for sociodemographic factors, men from Japanese, Korean, Chinese, South Asian, and Arab and West Asian backgrounds had earnings similar to white men.[1] However, Filipino,

Southeast Asian, Latin American, Black, and men from other marginalized groups earned significantly less, with the most significant disparities among Black and Latin American men. Even after accounting for employment characteristics like job type and occupation, Black, Latin American, and Filipino men still earned less than white men (Qiu and Schellenberg 2022, 17–18).

For women, only Black women earned significantly less than white women when sociodemographic factors were considered. In contrast, Chinese, South Asian, Filipina, and Southeast Asian women earned more than their white counterparts. Women in marginalized groups fared better relative to white women than minority men did (Qiu and Schellenberg 2022, 17–18).

Education plays a crucial role in these earnings gaps. Chinese and Korean individuals had university degrees 35–40% higher than white people, while South Asian and Japanese individuals had rates 20–25% higher. These educational advantages explain much of the earnings gaps for these groups. Conversely, Black and Latin American individuals had lower university degree rates, contributing to their earnings gaps (Qiu and Schellenberg 2022, 17–18).

Full-time jobs and higher paying occupations positively impacted earnings for Chinese, Korean, South Asian, and Japanese women, indicating that their educational qualifications led to better labour market outcomes. In contrast, part-time jobs and lower paying occupations negatively impacted the earnings of Black and Latin American men. From 2005 to 2015, earnings gaps for Black men and women and Latin American men widened, showing that these groups fell further behind over time (Qiu and Schellenberg 2022, 17–18). Race and gender alone cannot explain weekly earning differentials, as multiple factors shape wages and earnings.

Income and Poverty

Let us examine the extent of poverty in Canada and identify the most at-risk demographics.[2] Canada's official poverty line, the Market Basket Measure, showed that 10.3% of the population, roughly 4 million people, lived below the poverty line in 2019. The poverty rate dropped to 6.4% in 2020 (Statistics Canada 2023a, 6). This poverty reduction can be linked to income and social support provided by the government amidst the COVID-19 pandemic. However, in 2021, the poverty rate rose to 7.4%, impacting approximately 2.8 million people (Statistics Canada 2023a, 6). Why did this 1% increase occur? Part of the reason is that fewer people received government financial support in 2021 than in 2020.

Specifically, 16.1% of single-parent families lived in poverty in 2021. Breaking it down by gender, the poverty rate was higher in families headed by single females, at 17.2%, compared to families headed by single males, at 11.6% (Statistics Canada 2023a, 3), a difference of 5.6%. Poverty partly concerns employment income, family structure, and gender. So, if you are a single mother, you are more likely to experience poverty than a single father. Poverty is gendered.

Compared to non-racialized, racialized groups are more likely to be affected by poverty, regardless of gender. In 2021, while the overall poverty rate was 7.4%, the visible minority population had a poverty rate of 9.5% compared to 6.5% for the non-visible minority population. Specifically, 13.9% of Indigenous people aged 16 years and older lived in poverty. Similarly, higher percentages of Arab (12.8%), Chinese (11.7%), and Black (11.5%) individuals lived in poverty. Filipinos registered the lowest poverty rate, at 2.9% (Statistics Canada 2023a, 6).

Among the eleven racialized groups studied by Statistics Canada, ten had higher poverty rates than the white group. Some groups, such as South Asian and Japanese, had smaller gaps. In contrast, others like Arab, West Asian, and Korean had more significant disparities, even after adjusting for sociodemographic factors like sex, age, education, language, generational co-residence, household type, number of earners, population size, and geographic distribution (Schimmele et al. 2023, 5–16).

Compared to the white group, the South Asian group experienced slightly higher poverty rates in the first two generations, levelling off in the third and beyond. The Chinese and Japanese groups had higher poverty rates in the first generation, but these differences lessened in the second generation and reversed in the third and beyond. The Arab and Korean groups consistently had higher poverty rates, though the gaps were reduced with each generation. The Southeast Asian group maintained higher poverty rates across all generations, with a decrease from the first to the second generation but no further change in the third and beyond. The Black, Latin American, and West Asian groups had higher poverty rates in all generations, with declines from the first to the second generation; however, the most significant gaps appeared in the third and beyond. The Filipino group had a lower poverty rate than the white group across all generations (Schimmele et al. 2023, 5–16).

The Filipino group's lower poverty rate is primarily due to having more earners per household and higher education levels, which offset disadvantages related to immigrant status, language barriers, and age.

About 81% of the Filipino group lived in households with two or more earners, compared to 55% of the white group. This higher number of earners strongly correlates with lower poverty rates. If their sociodemographic profile were similar to the white group's, their poverty rate would be about one percentage point higher. These differences account for about 40% of the Filipino group's lower poverty rate compared to the white group (Schimmele et al. 2023, 5–16). Although lower in poverty percentage, the white group have more people experiencing poverty in absolute numbers because they comprise the largest segment of the population.

Poverty varies across ethnic groups, with some groups showing improvement over time and others maintaining higher rates compared to the white group. Driven by income and wealth distribution in capitalist societies, poverty is a primary cause of health inequities. Although intertwined with gender and race, it is fundamentally a class issue. Addressing poverty requires confronting the unequal class relations inherent in capitalism. To effectively address poverty, we need to unite those who are in poverty with individuals who have more economic stability but are still vulnerable within our capitalist system. These individuals are at risk of falling into poverty if they lose their jobs due to workplace closures or privatization. It is essential to acknowledge that certain groups experience higher poverty rates, but we should see them not as victims but as protagonists and capable workers facing unique but connected challenges. Solving these issues requires solidarity and a commitment to equality, involving collective efforts to remove the disadvantages faced by working-class members.

The State of Health Inequities

We worry about poverty, our jobs, where we live, and our health because they affect how long we live, how often we get sick, and how much we suffer. Although many people think Canada's health care system is excellent, we see pervasive health inequities. That is why finding better ways to make health fair for everyone is essential. This task is urgent, especially considering the unequal impacts of COVID-19 on those already experiencing health disadvantages.[3] Epidemiology, the study of how diseases spread and what causes them, is crucial for making policies that make people healthier and reduce health inequities. Using statistics to track how many people get sick or die from certain diseases, we can see where health problems are worse. The sections below show that Canada has many health inequities, and history has shown that we have not done a very good job of solving them.

Infant Mortality

The infant mortality rate is a health indicator that measures the number of deaths or the chance of dying within the first year of life per 1000 live births in a specific geographical area within a particular period. In Canada, the infant mortality rate steadily declined from 41.3/1000 in 1950 to 4.3/1000 in 2020 (Macrotrends n.d.a).[4] However, the improvement in the rate is unevenly distributed among the population. For instance, excluding Ontario due to unavailable data, the infant mortality rate for the lowest income group, representing 20% of the population, was 4.7/1000, while for the highest income group, representing the top 20% of the population, it was 3.2/1000 in 2008–11 (Government of Canada 2018a, 83). Generally, the lower the income, the higher the infant mortality rate.

In areas with a high concentration of Métis, First Nations, and Inuit populations, the infant mortality rate is 1.9, 2.3, and 3.9 times higher, respectively, compared to areas with lower concentrations of Indigenous Peoples. Regions with the lowest education levels have an infant mortality rate 1.6 times higher than those with the highest. Remote communities have a rate 1.5 times higher than large cities (Government of Canada 2018a, 77–86). Income is the primary determinant of uneven infant health outcomes, with education, ethnicity, and geography also playing significant roles. Addressing these interconnected social determinants of health is essential to ensuring infants have the best chance of being healthy.

Life Expectancy

The life expectancy at birth measures the population's overall mortality level. It tells us the average number of years a newborn will live considering the prevailing sex- and age-specific death rates at the time of their birth within a geographical area or country for a specific year (WHO n.d.). If we look at Canada, the life expectancy at birth has steadily increased over the years. In 1950, people in Canada were expected to live up to around 68 years on average. However, it had gone up to 82 years in 2020 (Macrotrends n.d.b).[5] This represents a gain to our life expectancy at birth of approximately 14 years since 1950.

At first glance, it seems people in Canada are healthier than those in many other countries, which is somewhat valid. However, when I dug deeper into the research and interviewed scholars, advocates, and activists, I uncovered a different story. There is substantial evidence that certain groups in Canada face health inequities due to social class, gender, and race, among other factors. In today's world, contentious debates about how class, gender, and race influence people's lives continue. In the health field, conflicting views on health inequalities based on class and other identities can make it hard to develop effective solutions. This issue is critical. While it is easier to study how class, gender, or race separately impact health, these power dynamics are integrally interconnected. Therefore, we need to understand how they all work together — how they are embedded — in our economic, political, cultural, and institutional systems to tackle health inequities more effectively.

Class–Health Axis

Throughout history, people experiencing poverty and those in the working class have suffered more illnesses and deaths compared to wealthy individuals and the capitalist class. In the nineteenth century, owners of factories that produced silk, cotton, and wool had workers labouring long hours for very little pay. This situation made it difficult for workers to afford necessities like food, housing, and clothing. These harsh working and living conditions led to serious health problems such as sleep deprivation, lung diseases, infections, injuries, and deaths from workplace accidents (Villermé [1840] 1988).

The impact of terrible working and living conditions was devastating for children living in households experiencing poverty. For example, about half of the children born to cotton factory workers died before they were 2 years old. Meanwhile, children born to factory bosses and business owners lived up to 29 years longer than their workers (Villermé [1840] 1988, 36). This significant 27-year difference in life expectancy demonstrates how economic inequality, driven by unequal class relations, results in unfair health outcomes.

In 1842, Edwin Chadwick significantly impacted our understanding of health, arguing that people were dying from contagious diseases like fever, typhus, smallpox, and measles, as well as from lung, brain, nerve, and digestive diseases, primarily due to living conditions. These conditions, including unsanitary houses, inadequate drainage, and dangerous surroundings, led to vast differences in health. For example, people on one street lived 15 years on average, while those on the next street lived 60 years (Chadwick 1842, 83), a 45-year difference in life expectancy! Chadwick suggested that improving housing, drainage, and ventilation would make people healthier. He argued that the government could implement these changes by passing laws. While his policy ideas were practical, Chadwick did not fully understand how class relations affect health inequities. It is essential to realize that achieving fair health means more than just fixing housing and environmental problems. We also need to address inequalities caused by capitalism.

Let us consider the work of famous social epidemiologists in the twentieth century. For example, Richard Wilkinson showed that joblessness and wage gaps create income inequality among social classes, which affects health. He argued that people generally live longer in developed nations, where income and wealth are more equal. However, in countries with less social cohesion, income gaps are more significant, and low-income people experience more illnesses and die earlier than wealthy people (Wilkinson 1989, 1992, 1997). Nevertheless, while discussing social unity, many epidemiologists forget to account for how politics and power relations based on antagonistic class conflicts affect health (Muntaner and Lynch 1999). Like Chadwick, they often do not consider how unequal class relations might explain why some people are sicker than others. They do not discuss how the imbalance of power relations among owners, bosses, and workers worsens health inequities.

Startling data regarding the early days of the COVID-19 pandemic reveals vast inequalities in income and health. For example, in June 2020, in Toronto, households earning less than $29,999 per year made up 31% of all COVID-19 cases, even though they comprised only 14% of the population. Meanwhile, households making over $150,000 a year, which comprised 21% of the population, had only 7% of COVID-19 cases (City of Toronto n.d.). Immigrants, people without legal status, and those with insecure jobs faced even more financial and health problems (Borras, Goldring, and Landolt 2021). The pandemic brought many pressing problems, with lockdowns and economic troubles hitting hard on people with low wages, those living in poverty, and members of marginalized groups.

Our story demonstrates how class relations and subsequent wealth distribution create health inequities. The evidence clearly shows the gaps between wealthy capitalists and impoverished workers. One key point is that capitalists — regardless of their race or gender — always seek more profit and keep wages low for workers. As a result, many workers earn too little, trapping their families in a cycle of poverty: living in inadequate housing and struggling to get enough nutritious food and access to health services. Capitalism produces vast health gaps between rich and poor; working-class families have higher rates of death, disease, and illness compared to the capitalist class.

Class–Gender–Health Axis

Understanding that social relations are complex and involve multiple factors is crucial. While women generally live longer than men, this is not always the case when comparing high-income countries and low-income countries. Even within a single country, women in poverty experience more morbidities and higher mortality rates than wealthy men. This health inequality is partly due to gender bias and discrimination. For example, many family doctors do not take women's complaints, such as headaches or tiredness, as seriously as they do men's (Armitage et al. 1979). Psychiatrists prescribe more mood-altering drugs to women because they assume women are emotionally unstable (Aggleton 1990). Health inequalities also affect reproductive health (Gielen et al. 1994). In the past, male doctors restricted midwives from performing medical and surgical procedures during childbirth (Ehrenreich and English 1973).

Male power continues to cause domestic violence, which includes mental, physical, and sexual abuse, leading to a condition called battered woman syndrome (Clark 2011). Gender violence also results in malnutrition, forced isolation, infectious diseases, and deaths (Laurie and Petchesky 2008). These health inequities based on gender arise from beliefs and narratives that favour straight men over women and other genders.[6]

However, gender relations are not separate from other social relations. Gender and class relations are integrally entwined, especially in occupational settings. For instance, in the nineteenth century, women, children, and men all suffered from harsh working conditions. Even young girls and older women had to perform strenuous work for long hours with lower wages than men. Driven by capital accumulation, capitalists did not care about the health of workers and their families as long as they made a profit. Capitalists generally viewed women, girls, children, the elderly, and persons with disabilities as less productive and therefore less profitable than able-bodied adult men, resulting in them typically receiving lower wages for performing the same labour.

Two centuries later, in patriarchal capitalist workplaces, women continue to experience preventable adverse health outcomes related to employment and working conditions:

> Women suffer many problems related to their work: musculoskeletal problems from repetitive work, constrained work postures, overuse, and tools and work sites ill-adapted

to their size and shape; stress leading to heart disease and psychological distress from multiple demands, sexual and sexist harassment, lack of job control, emotion work and job demands incompatible with pregnancy, nursing and family life; cancers, skin disease and toxic effects of chemical exposures such as those in hairdressing, factory work, hospitals, laboratories, cleaning and farm work; reproductive problems such as dysmenorrhea, irregular cycles and difficult pregnancies associated with exposures to chemicals, ergonomic stresses and difficult work schedules; violence from clients and co-workers; eyestrain from meticulous work and the requirement to work without error, and exhaustion from overwork, inadequate rest breaks and repetitive work. (Messing and de Grosbois 2001, 126)

Gendered health inequities at work continue because of sexist practices and rules in the workplace (Armstrong and Armstrong 2003; Morrow et al. 2007; Syed et al. 2016; Syed and Ahmad 2021), which are part of how the capitalist system uses and controls workers. By working together, feminists, labour groups, scientists, and researchers can better tackle these problems (Messing and de Grosbois 2001). The struggles of women in workplaces and other male-dominated spaces reflect the challenges that many women and girls face worldwide.

Globally, 2,153 billionaires, primarily white heterosexual males, possess wealth exceeding that of 4.6 billion people worldwide. Part of this wealth gap arises from the uncompensated work that women and girls contribute to the world's economy, worth approximately $11 trillion annually (Coffey et al. 2020, 8). The root cause of this vast gendered inequity is the "sexist economic system that values the wealth of the privileged few, mostly men, more than the billions of hours of the essential work — the unpaid and underpaid care work done primarily by women and girls around the world" (2). As a result, women and girls face greater poverty risk.

Gender-based poverty — shaped by capitalism — results in unequal health outcomes. Women worldwide, because of poverty, are more likely to face problems like depression, communicable diseases, malnutrition, and cancer. They also have less access to health services than men (Doyal 1995). Women and girls, devalued by capitalist societies, rarely participate in decision-making processes in public and private spaces dominated by men. The sexism that favours straight men also harms non-straight men, affecting their work, living conditions, and health. We must address health inequities caused by intricately interconnected class and gender dynamics.

Class–Race–Health Axis

In the past, European countries took over other lands to exploit their resources and people. Colonized peoples endured the triple burden of economic exploitation, political repression, and cultural-racial discrimination, shaping health inequities. This history of colonization affects how groups and classes relate today in workplaces, neighbourhoods, and governments. Ideas and practices from colonial times continue to make life unfair for Indigenous Peoples and people from former colonies, resulting in health inequities. Although there is limited research directly connecting public and population health to colonialism, there is ample evidence showing that health inequities based on race, ethnicity, and Indigeneity exist today.

Even before COVID-19, we saw how race and class relations impacted health. Unfair medical practices in Western capitalist societies resulted in people receiving different treatments for heart problems based on their race (Fincher et al. 2004). Pregnant people and people needing mental health care struggled to get the help they needed because of racism (Kirby, Taliaferro, and Zuvekas 2006). Racism even led to more babies dying (Wallace et al. 2017). A review of 333 articles shows that racism, especially when linked to socioeconomic problems, adversely impacts health in numerous ways (Paradies et al. 2015). Specifically, racialized poverty results in disparities in rates of diabetes (Chaufan, Davis, and Constantino 2011). Health inequities arise from structural racism, which is institutionalized in capitalist societies.[7]

The COVID-19 pandemic further revealed how the combined impact of racism and colonial histories affects health outcomes. Early pandemic data clearly showed growing health gaps among racialized groups. This inequality arose because some people have better access to basic needs, such as suitable housing, sufficient nutritious food, and affordable health services than others.

In May 2020, the Navajo Nation had a higher COVID-19 infection rate than New Jersey and New York. We can link the infection rate variances to the fact that despite lockdowns, many people in the Navajo Nation live in overcrowded housing, making it difficult to escape the spread of the virus between household members. Moreover, many households do not have access to clean running water, making hygiene practices challenging. Lastly, the Navajo Nation is a food desert (Silverman et al. 2020), meaning people have limited access to an adequate supply of nutritious food. Capitalist settler-colonialism continues to marginalize Indigenous communities, increasing their vulnerability to illnesses and deaths.

In the US, compared to white non-Hispanics, Asians were 1.3 times, Hispanics or Latinos 4.6 times, African Americans 4.7 times, and Indigenous people 5.3 times more likely to be hospitalized due to COVID-19 in August 2020 (Centers for Disease Control and Prevention n.d.). These numbers show that Indigenous people faced the highest risk of COVID-19 hospitalizations, while white non-Hispanics faced the least risk. Another sad truth is that while 26 out of every 100,000 white non-Hispanics died from the virus, the numbers were higher for minority groups: 66 for African Americans, 32 for Indigenous people, 30 for Hispanics or Latinos, and 28 for Asians in July 2020 (COVID Tracking Project n.d.).[8]

In Ontario, COVID-19 hit hard in marginalized neighbourhoods. These areas, with more immigrants and racialized groups, have low incomes, high poverty levels, insecure housing, and a lack of basic resources. People who died from COVID-19 were more likely to live in these places (Chung et al. 2020). It is obvious that some racial and ethnic groups were getting hit harder, with non-white communities having more COVID-19 cases, hospitalizations, and deaths. These inequities result from past colonialism and ongoing racism built into capitalist societies where colonized and racialized groups are economically exploited and oppressed at the same time.

Class-Gender-Race-Health Axis

We have explored how different social systems influence the health of individuals, families, and communities. Now, consider someone who has an unstable job, is struggling to make ends meet, and is a woman of a visibly non-white ethnicity. Her experiences with living, working, and health will be very different from those of people from other backgrounds. This is why it is crucial to examine how class, gender, and race relations collectively create health inequities.

Having little money or being poor means one might not have enough food. People who cannot afford nutritious food experience food insecurity, malnutrition, and hunger. In 2022, around 2.4 billion people, or one-third of the world's population, did not always have enough food; about 900 million faced severe food insecurity (FAO et al. 2023, 7). Reports show a surge in food insecurity in Canada, with the number of individuals affected rising from 5.8 million in 2020 to 6.9 million in 2021 (Statistics Canada 2023a, 4), an increase of 1.1 million people. This is due to a decrease in government financial aid and an increase in fuel and food prices. Despite Canada's wealth, millions still struggle with food insecurity. People experiencing food insecurity face a higher risk of developing adverse health conditions, including diabetes, hypertension, heart disease, mood disorders, depression, anxiety, migraines, stomach ulcers, bowel disorders, back problems, and arthritis (Tarasuk et al. 2013), contributing to early deaths. Alarmingly, death rates for severely, moderately, and marginally food-insecure individuals were approximately 160%, 49%, and 28% higher, respectively, than for food-secure individuals (Gundersen et al. 2018, 6).

Who is most likely to face food insecurity and its adverse health outcomes? In Canada, as of 2021, around 52% of households struggling with food insecurity relied on incomes from wages, salaries, or self-employment (Tarasuk et al. 2022, 19). These statistics show that class relations between the capitalists and workers and socioeconomic status significantly shape food insecurity. Racial dynamics also play a crucial role in food insecurity. While the food insecurity rate for people not in racialized groups was 16%, lower than the national average of 18.4%, there are stark differences: 31% of Indigenous people off-reserve, 39% of Black individuals, 29% of Filipinos, 27% of Arabs, 22% of Southeast Asians, 21% of South Asians, 20% of Latin Americans, and 18% of Chinese individuals faced food insecurity in 2021 (Statistics Canada 2023a, 7). This data illustrates that the financial reasons behind food insecurity are intertwined with Indigeneity, race, and ethnicity.

Furthermore, gender dynamics contribute to food insecurity, especially for families with children. In 2021, 21% of persons living in couple families with children experienced food insecurity. In the same year, out of the additional 1.1 million individuals experiencing food insecurity, 802,000 were from families with children. Single-parent families headed by women had a higher rate of food insecurity, at 43%, compared to 24% in single-parent families headed by men (Statistics Canada 2023a, 4–7). Women-led single-parent families are nearly twice as likely to face food insecurity as those led by men.

Food insecurity, similar to poverty, impacts groups differently, primarily due to differences in class, race, gender, and family status. Notably, low-income racialized single mothers face a higher risk of health issues and premature death because they struggle to buy enough healthy food.

Food insecurity is a complex problem, highlighting how social relations are inherently interconnected, with social class — poverty — being the core determining factor of food insecurity, whether it is racialized or gendered food insecurity.

Throughout this book, we examine how social relations shape resource distribution, leading to inequalities in wealth and power based on class, gender, and race, which, in turn, create health disparities. These disparities are not natural; they arise from societal systems established by human beings. Therefore, we can change them. To address health inequities, we must take bold steps to challenge and transform the current state of affairs.

Notes

1. I chose this study because it uniquely examines sociodemographic factors, such as job type, occupation, and education, impacting weekly earnings for Canadian-born workers aged 25 to 44, based on the 2016 Census and published in 2022. While newer data on weekly earnings by race exist, it does not account for these specific factors.
2. Tables can be found in Statistics Canada 2023a. See also Schimmele et al. 2023.
3. Rob Wallace (2020) and Wallace et al. (2020) assert that recent pandemics, such as MERS, SARS, and COVID-19, are consequences of the global capitalist industrial food system's destruction of ecological balance.
4. For graphs and tables, access "Canada Infant Mortality Rate 1950–2024" (Macrotrends n.d.a).
5. Graphs and tables can be accessed via the "Canada Life Expectancy 1950–2024" (Macrotrends n.d.b).
6. Heteropatriarchal sexism is a system where heterosexual, cisgender men hold most of the power in society. It is composed of two main ideas: that being attracted to the opposite gender is the norm and that men should dominate in all parts of life. This system supports male power, traditional ideas about relationships, and separate roles for men and women (Kelley and Arce-Trigatti 2021; Valdes 1996). The inequalities resulting from these beliefs lead to unfair societal situations, negatively affecting people's health.
7. Race influences resource distribution and social relations, impacting activism and anti-racist strategies (Hall 1997/2021). Originally used to justify biological divisions, race is now a social construct creating hierarchies with whiteness at the top, leading to marginalization and atrocities. *Racialization* assigns significance to race, categorizing groups as unequal and stigmatizing traits linked to racialized groups, perpetuating inequality and privileging whites (NCCDH 2018; OHRC 2005). *Racism* promotes inequality through stereotypes, prejudice, and discrimination, benefiting whites and disadvantaging minorities (Berman and Paradies 2010; McGibbon 2021). It operates on multiple levels: internalized racism (belief group superiority or inferiority), interpersonal-individual racism

(subtle interactions that can lead to job loss for example), systemic-institutional racism (institutional policies causing inequalities), and societal-structural racism (cultural ideologies permeating society) (Berman and Paradies, 2010; NCCDH 2018; OHRC 2005). Racism perpetuates systemic inequalities and racialized health inequities through individual beliefs, interpersonal interactions, institutional policies, and societal norms.

8   The author retrieved these early-stage pandemic data from The COVID Tracking Project's COVID Racial Data Tracker on July 12, 2020. They provide insights into states' preparedness during emergencies. The most recent data, published on March 7, 2021, is accessible at https://covidtracking.com/race.

CHAPTER TWO

Neoliberalism and Canada's Housing Policies

Politics and economics are deeply connected, and there are three main ways to examine how money and political power affect health: (1) neoclassical economics, or microeconomics; (2) Keynesian economics, or macroeconomics; and (3) Marxist economics. *Neoclassical economics* ties individual well-being to consuming goods and services, suggesting that more consumption leads to greater well-being. It views capitalism — with its principles of individual freedom, private property, and market exchanges — as the ideal society, producing maximum output and consumption while balancing profits and individual needs. Neoclassical economics focuses on market interactions among individuals (e.g., buyers and sellers) and advocates for less government involvement, trusting that competition will resolve issues like poverty, housing, and health care (Wolff and Resnick 2012, 51–104). In short, neoclassical economics emphasizes individual consumption and market competition with minimal state intervention to address socioeconomic and health inequities.

The Great Depression of the 1930s exposed the limits of neoclassical economics, showing that free markets could not prevent the collapse of capitalism. The capitalist class saw a social revolution from the unemployed, the poor, and those disillusioned with capitalism as the immediate threat. To rescue capitalism, economist John Maynard Keynes proposed monetary and fiscal policies to ensure employment, price stability, and economic growth.[1] Keynes viewed the economy as a network of social relationships influencing individual behaviour. *Keynesian economics* focuses on national employment rates and wealth distribution, and their impact on society and health. It advocates for extensive government intervention to address capitalism's imperfections, including economic depressions, forming the basis of "state-managed capitalism" (Wolff and Resnick 2012,

105–32). This approach supports equitable policies such as full employment, poverty alleviation, public housing, and health care access.

Marxist economics emphasizes the significance of class and labour exploitation, arguing that these dynamics fundamentally shape perceptions and actions, leading to social conflict and revolution. Marxists assert that capitalists exploit workers to maximize profit and consolidate power. Unlike proponents of neoclassical and Keynesian economists, who aim to reform and improve capitalism, Marxists seek to replace it with socialism through class struggle (Wolff and Resnick 2012, 133–250). They contend that socialism can effectively address socioeconomic and health inequities, which are inherent in capitalism.

The influence of these economic theories and practices oscillates over time. From the 1870s to 1914, neoclassical economics dominated, relegating Marxist economics to trade unions and socialist parties. However, between 1914 and 1945, significant events elevated the prominence of Marxist economics. The devastation of two world wars led many to blame capitalism for the turmoil. The 1917 Russian Revolution established a Marxist government, and the Union of Soviet Socialist Republics' rapid industrialization, attributed to Marxism, garnered global attention. The Great Depression also discredited capitalism, paving the way for Keynesian economics, which temporarily supplanted neoclassical economics from the 1940s to the 1970s (Wolff and Resnick 2012, 310–45).

The economic collapse of the 1930s led to state-interventionist capitalism, shifting economic practice toward Keynesian economics. Keynesianism introduced policies addressing money supply, interest rates, taxation, and spending. However, the crises of the 1970s, including the oil crisis and stagflation, prompted a shift back to deregulated capitalism, championed by leaders like Thatcher, Reagan, and Mulroney. During this period, Eastern European economies transitioned from state to private capitalism (Wolff and Resnick 2012, 310–45).

The 1980s and 1990s saw a further decline in the power of workers and people's movements, including socialist parties, resulting in a global shift toward reduced state roles in capitalism. These developments restored neoclassical economics to dominance, relegating Keynesian and Marxian economics to secondary positions and leading to the intensification of "private (often called 'neoliberal') forms of capitalism" (Wolff and Resnick 2012, 310–45). These shifts illustrate the dynamic nature of economic thought and its responsiveness to historical events, reflecting the changing dynamics and crises of capitalism.[2]

Neoliberalism

Neoliberalism, rooted in liberal principles, emphasizes free markets, private ownership, and individual freedoms. Unlike classical liberalism, which advocates for minimal government involvement in societal affairs, neoliberalism actively employs the state mechanisms to promote capital interests through policymaking (see John and P.M. 2019). Emerging in the late 1930s, neoliberalism gained traction by the mid-twentieth century, bolstered by right-wing think tanks and corporations. A shift from Keynesian to neoliberal policy approaches occurred in the 1970s (Harvey 2007, 9–19). This radical shift was catalyzed by economic challenges such as stagflation — a period characterized by stagnant growth, high unemployment, and soaring inflation.

By the 1980s, US-dominated global financial institutions, including the International Monetary Fund and World Bank, intensified the imposition of neoliberal adjustment policies, which largely benefited elites and capitalists rather than the masses, including workers. Neoliberalism influences four key areas of social life — economics, politics, culture, and institutions — that significantly impact individual, family, and community health. To better understand health inequities, it is crucial to grasp how neoliberalism operates in these fields.

Economic/Financial Sphere

After World War II, the Keynesian approach aspired to improve the lives of working-class people by rebalancing economic wealth and power. However, it was easily weakened since it did not fully replace core capitalist ideas and practices. By the 1970s, large corporations, feeling their power slipping, pushed for neoliberal state policies to regain control. This policy shift was a deliberate strategy against the rising power of the working class (Harvey 2005, 2007). Neoliberalism's success gave Big Capital more wealth and power,[3] leading to greater economic inequalities, political imbalances, cultural divisions, institutional conflicts, environmental harms, and health inequities.

The US Empire used global financial organizations to force countries to follow neoliberal rules, including cutting public spending, making trade easier, allowing industries to do what they wanted, and selling off government-owned businesses. These policies strengthened neoliberalism and maintained its heavy influence on economic and political activities. The shift from Keynesian to neoliberal policies demonstrates the constant battle between different classes and countries for wealth, power, and domination.

Political/Legal Sphere

Neoliberalism is not just about economics; it is also a political reaction to the growing power of the working class in democracies. When workers gained more rights and prevented excessive capital accumulation, big businesses saw it as a threat to making more profit. So, they pushed for neoliberal policies, which weakened workers' democratic gains and institutions. This political action reflects an ongoing fight between democratic values and the power of big money (Panitch and Gindin 2004, 2). Neoliberalism ensures that Big Capital stays in charge while pushing back against workers' interests.

Cultural/Ideological Sphere

Neoliberalism encompasses not only economic and political dimensions but also a cultural dimension. This ideology, embraced by the global elite, worsens health disparities by favouring the rich and capitalists in state policies. These policies benefit big businesses by making it easier for companies to fire workers through downsizing tactics, allowing big banks to operate with minimal restrictions, establishing trade rules that hurt workers and farmers, cutting funding for social programs, privatizing services, promoting consumerism and selfishness, praising the market while concealing the extent of collusion between businesses and governments, and advocating for government non-intervention while facilitating the satisfaction of the interests of the wealthy and capitalist class (Navarro 2007a). Neoliberalism impacts health and exacerbates health inequities (Labonté and Stuckler 2015; Navarro 2007b; Schrecker 2016; Scott-Samuel et al. 2014). Neoliberalism keeps big money and influential people on top, leaving others behind.

Institutional Sphere

But neoliberalism goes beyond cultural, economic, and political ideas. It is a complicated system with processes shaping public policies and people's beliefs. It is not just about how workers and businesses interact or what people think about capitalism. It affects everything from how the economy works to how people live and think about the world around them. Different groups, organizations, and institutions respond to neoliberalism differently — some like it, some fight against it, and some ignore it. This dynamic leads to significant changes in society (Hall and Lamont 2013). Neoliberalism does not only impact health policies; it affects everything in society and makes businesses, governments, civil society groups, and ordinary people react differently.

Neoliberalism promotes privatization and prioritizes the interests of capitalists in state policies. It advocates for more open trade that benefits rich nations and influential individuals over poorer nations and the general populace. Neoliberal policies swing between loosening rules for businesses to allow bigger profits and imposing stricter rules for workers, constraining wages and benefits. When governments cut back on spending, it harms low-income people the most. Capitalism limits the influence of workers and ordinary people on state decisions impacting societal and public health affairs. In neoliberalism, the close relationship between big businesses and the government means policies mostly favour capital power and interests. This strong alliance between capital and the state prevents housing policies with socialist ideas from addressing housing-related health inequities.

Historicizing Canada's Housing Policies

In the past, our government mainly responded to housing issues during disasters, strikes, or economic crashes. Eventually, the government started focusing on creating a welfare system to help people who needed it. This policy shift led to more organized efforts to provide housing for struggling individuals, families, and communities, thereby improving their well-being. From the mid-1930s to the 1950s, significant changes occurred in Canada's housing policy. In 1935, Prime Minister Bennett's government initiated a program offering affordable mortgages to middle-income homebuyers. Subsequently, in 1938, King's government introduced public housing and financed local agencies for its construction. During World War II, a government agency provided housing for veterans and workers. After the war, another government agency managed these homes (McInnes 1987, 1–12). This period demonstrates how the state and its apparatuses utilized housing policy to stimulate the economy and address housing challenges during difficult times, particularly by meeting the urgent demand to house the influx of workers flocking to urban centres for wartime production.

In the mid-1940s, more programs for affordable housing were initiated. Notable projects such as Benny Farm in Montreal and Regent Park in Toronto provided subsidized and public housing. In 1949, amendments to the National Housing Act established the Public Housing Program, in which the federal government contributed 75% of the housing costs, with provinces and territories (PTs) covering the remainder. This policy focused on housing provisions for low-income families, people with disabilities, and older adults (CMHC 2011, 128–31). After World War II, there was a significant increase in public housing construction, leading to a housing boom. This era witnessed extensive state involvement in affordable housing, reflecting a broader trend toward government intervention in housing policy to address socioeconomic inequalities and political upheavals.

In the 1960s, housing cooperatives gained popularity. Willow Park Housing Cooperative in Manitoba, founded in 1966, was the first cooperative designed for families, and its success led to the creation of the Cooperative Housing Federation of Canada. The National Labour Cooperatives Committee, supported by the Canadian Labour Congress and the Cooperative Union of Canada, played a crucial role in this endeavour. Abbotsford Co-op was the first cooperative for older adults, while De Cosmos Village Cooperative aided low-income families. In 1969, citizens in Vancouver initiated the first housing renovation project, the Strathcona Project (CMHC 2011, 131–33). These cooperatives, managed by their residents and with solid support from labour unions, shifted away from individual homeownership to communal ownership.

The Pierre Trudeau government introduced four new housing programs in 1973–74: (1) the Cooperative Housing Program offered long-term mortgages to support cooperative housing developments; (2) the Non-Profit Housing Program provided rental housing for families with moderate to low incomes, with support from community groups; (3) the Rent Supplement Program assisted low-income tenants by lowering their monthly rent based on their income; and (4) the Rural and Native Housing Program was initiated to address the needs of low-income families in small rural communities (CMHC 2011, 133–35).

While the ruling governments focused on providing affordable housing through public and community housing programs from the 1930s, in the 1970s, they started favouring neoliberal policies, which meant reducing the housing budget allocation. This policy change made it harder for people to find stable housing, resulting in more insecurity and homelessness. From the 1980s to the 1990s, state policies further intensified neoliberal ideas. Specifically, after the Progressive Conservative Party won the 1984 election, the Mulroney government drastically reduced housing and social supports. Then, in 1986, the Urban Native Housing Program was incorporated into a larger Social Housing Strategy (CMHC 2011, 136). By 1993, the government had cut nearly $2 billion in funding for housing, and there were no new social housing projects (Bryant and Raphael 2020, 70).

After winning the 1993 election, the Liberal Party made more cuts to housing support, with the Chrétien government eliminating national social housing programs. In 1996, the federal government shifted housing responsibilities to local governments through the Social Housing Agreements. These policy changes caused significant problems with housing, resulting in the United Nations becoming involved in addressing Canada's severe housing insecurity and homelessness issues (United Nations 1999). The federal government responded to this harsh criticism by launching the National Homelessness Initiative in 2000 and the Affordable Housing Initiative in 2001. These programs required contributions from both the public and private sectors. Furthermore, after the Conservative Party won in 2006, the Harper government created the Northern Housing Trust and the Affordable Housing Trust to address housing problems during the global financial crisis (CMHC 2011, 137–38). During this period, the government only stepped in to address housing issues after problems arose rather than acting beforehand. So, the state's housing policy is reactive, not proactive.

In April 2007, the National Homelessness Initiative was renamed the Homelessness Partnering Strategy (HPS). However, by November 2007, the UN Special Rapporteur on Affordable Housing reported that Canada was facing a twin crisis of housing insecurity and homelessness (United Nations 2007). This rebuke prompted the government to change its policies, and in 2008, they provided $110 million over five years for the At Home/Chez Soi research project (Goering et al. 2014, 6). This project introduced the "Housing First" approach to dealing with homelessness and mental health issues.[4]

In the 2010s, Canada's housing policy saw substantial investments. For example, the government committed $1.4 billion to the Affordable Housing 2011–14 Framework Agreement (Homeless Hub n.d.), and the HPS was extended until 2019. The 2015 federal election brought the Liberal Party to power, leading to the National Housing Strategy (NHS), announcement in November 2017. This landmark policy was in response to a reprimand by the UN Committee on Economic and Social Rights about poverty, housing insecurity, and homelessness in the country (United Nations 2016). Notably, domestic actions and critiques from the UN have prompted the federal government to focus more on these interrelated issues.

The NHS is a significant project, with $40 billion set aside for ten years. Its goal is to make major improvements in housing by (1) removing 530,000 households from core housing need, (2) repairing 300,000 units, (3) building 100,000 new units, (4) keeping 385,000 community housing units safe, (5) helping 300,000 households with the Canada Housing Benefit, and (6) reducing chronic homelessness by 50% by 2028 (Government of Canada 2018b, 4–7). The NHS emphasizes collaboration among governments, businesses, and non-profit organizations for its implementation. In 2019, the National Housing Strategy Act was legislated, embedding a human rights approach to housing. It also mandated the National Housing Council to make policies that include everyone.

At present, it is difficult to evaluate how well the NHS works because of the ongoing effects of the COVID-19 pandemic. Additionally, when the Bank of Canada repeatedly raised interest rates, it delivered more money to the big real estate owners at the expense of the middle-class, low-income earners and those experiencing poverty. Even with the NHS, more people are struggling with housing, and millions are relying on food banks.

The Impact of Neoliberal Housing Policies

Around the world, neoliberal programs have resulted in over a billion people living in slums (Davis 2017, 23). In wealthier countries, there was rampant privatization of social housing units. This policy seemed beneficial, allowing low-income people to become homeowners, but it did not turn out that way. Instead, housing prices soared, and original residents who could not afford the higher prices were forced to move to poorer areas of the cities. Neighbourhoods where working-class people lived started getting fancier, which made housing less secure and led to more homelessness (Harvey 2005, 157–69). Even though it seemed like aiding people, selling off public housing and pushing for private ownership harmed many of them, making their lives worse.

In big cities like Toronto, gentrification significantly changes neighbourhoods and communities. This urban and housing development is happening in areas like South Riverdale and Leslieville. In these places, average incomes increased by 47%, from $70,000 to over $103,000, and average house prices went up from $320,000 to $765,000 between 2006 and 2015. In Dovercourt-Wallace Emerson, the Junction, and Trinity Bellwoods, incomes rose even more, by an average of 53%, compared to just an 18% increase in Toronto overall. Unfortunately, while about 22% of neighbourhoods showed signs of gentrification, only 0.4% of households went from low-income to high-income (King 2016), meaning that lower income people are forced out of neighbourhoods while higher income people are moving in. Gentrification is not only about making real estate more valuable; it underscores how capitalism perpetuates inequalities. Gentrification is not just about how a city looks — it is about who can afford and cannot afford to live there. Regent Park, Lawrence Heights, and Parkdale are neighbourhoods where gentrification is also a big issue. In Parkdale, big international real estate companies are buying up the houses, causing more people to be displaced and mistreated. Long-time residents are trying to fight against these changes, but newer immigrants who do not know their rights well are leaving quietly (Whyte 2020). The shift from local landlords to big companies shows that profit is the main reason behind these changes. Gentrification goes beyond housing itself; it is a capitalist strategy for more extensive economic change and sustained capital accumulation.

Gentrification also occurs in Brooklyn, San Francisco, London, Berlin, and other major cities worldwide. It primarily satisfies the needs of corporations, making housing more expensive and raising living costs. Gentrification fuels economic growth, but it widens inequalities. To understand how it affects communities and people with limited financial resources, we must look at it closely and try to make city development more fair and healthy for everyone.

Neoliberal housing policies have caused the following problems: (1) housing prices keep rising faster than people's earnings; (2) converting cheaper apartments into expensive condos has made it much harder to find affordable housing; (3) rents keep increasing, making it difficult for millions to afford housing; and (4) the government's termination of public housing support worsened the housing situation (Hulchanski et al. 2009; Pomeroy 2015). These problems affect low-income workers, single-parent families headed by women, and people from racialized communities more than other classes and groups.

Neoliberal housing policies have made housing insecurity and homelessness much worse in recent years. Before these policies, people in Canada did not see homelessness as a social and health problem. However, since the 1980s, visible homelessness has become widespread (Hulchanski et al. 2009, 1–16), exacerbating health inequities.[5] Unsurprisingly, in 2022, Toronto Public Health found that men who are experiencing homelessness die at age 55 and women at age 42. This is way younger than the average age of death in Toronto, which is 79 for men and 84 for women (City of Toronto 2023). Being homeless thus shortens life expectancy by about 24 years for men and 42 years for women! Homelessness is a grave injustice against humanity.

Housing insecurity and homelessness occur because the state and its agencies support real estate and banking corporations that continuously increase housing prices. This setup is a huge problem because these entities focus on generating profit and capital accumulation. The Greenbelt Scandal in Ontario revealed how the government made decisions that served the interests of big companies instead of the public (McGrath 2023; Office of the Auditor General of Ontario 2023). This scandal is an example of neoliberalism and a corrupt style of governance (Moscrop 2023). We need to stop using neoliberal strategies and focus on socialized housing.

Neoliberalism and the State of Housing Insecurity

In Canada, the term "core housing need" refers to households, either individuals or families, that cannot meet specific housing standards. This concept is crucial for understanding the link between housing policy, housing insecurity, and public health. The Canada Mortgage and Housing Corporation defines this need based on *affordability* (housing costs exceeding 30% of pre-tax income), *suitability* (housing condition and need for repairs), and *adequacy* (sufficient bedrooms for all members). A household failing to meet any of these standards is in core housing need (CMHC 2018, 2-1). This book uses "core housing need" and "housing insecurity" interchangeably, emphasizing that housing insecurity results from unmet affordability, suitability, and adequacy standards.

Housing Insecurity and Health

Poor-quality housing harms our physical, mental, and psychosocial health. Substandard housing leads to more sickness and deaths among low-income workers and people experiencing poverty. In the 1800s, working-class housing in the cities — constructed for profit and capital accumulation — caused the proliferation of city slums (Engels 1845, 85). This issue, where capitalism creates inhumane living conditions, remains a significant problem today. Living in slums extends beyond lacking space and basic amenities; it is a global health crisis. In Manila's slums, the infant mortality rate was three times higher than the city's average (Fry, Cousins, and Olivola 2002, xiii). In Quito, slum areas had an infant mortality rate thirty times higher than wealthier areas (Stephens 1996, 16). Similar patterns exist in Nairobi and Dhaka slums, where children face much higher mortality rates compared to those in non-slum areas (Herr and Karl 2002; Mberu et al. 2016).

In Mumbai, slum mortality rates were 50% higher than in nearby rural areas (Davis 2017, 146). Even in Canada, slums pose serious challenges. There is no doubt that housing insecurity affects health. The World Health Organization (2018) warns that poor housing causes stress, breathing problems, injuries, infectious diseases, and heart issues. The COVID-19 pandemic has worsened these issues, especially in slums, where it is hard to maintain physical distance. These living conditions violate fundamental human rights to housing, health, and life. Living in slums is a humanitarian crisis.

The Housing Insecure

Data from CMHC brings housing insecurity in Canada and who it affects into focus.[6] Between 2001 and 2016, even though the percentage of insecure households decreased, the number of insecure households increased. In 2001, around 1.5 million households (14%) experienced housing insecurity, rising to 1.7 million (13%) in 2016 (CMHC 2020a, 2020b). This trend means there were over 200,000 more insecure households during this period.

Housing insecurity predominantly affects renters. In 2001, over 1.0 million renter households and 470,000 homeowner households were housing insecure. By 2016, these numbers rose to about 1.1 million renters and 574,000 homeowners (CMHC 2020a, 2020b), indicating an increase of 100,000 for renters and 104,000 for homeowners over fifteen years. In 2001, 28.3% of renters and 6.6% of homeowners faced housing insecurity. In 2016, these rates slightly decreased to 26.8% for renters and 6.3% for homeowners (CMHC 2020a, 2020b). Notably, despite the decrease in percentages, the number of affected households increased significantly, with renters nearly four times more likely to face housing insecurity than homeowners.

Class and Housing Insecurity

Housing insecurity has escalated, especially for households allocating over 30% of their income to housing. From 2001 to 2016, households falling below the affordability standard increased from about one million to 1.28 million, marking an overall increase of over 280,000 households in fifteen years. Homeowners saw a greater increase than renters, with about 114,000 more homeowners and 105,000 more renters affected (CMHC 2020a, 2020b). This trend is mainly due to housing costs rising faster than income growth.

Gender and Housing Insecurity

Gender affects housing insecurity, especially for single-parent families. In 2016, there were over 307,000 single-parent families who struggled with housing, and most of them, about 266,000, were led by women. In contrast, only about 40,000 were led by men (CMHC 2020b). Among renters who faced housing insecurity, roughly 198,000 households were led by women, compared to only 26,000 by men. For homeowners who struggled with housing insecurity, around 69,000 were led by women, while only 15,000 were led by men (CMHC 2020b). These numbers highlight that compared to male-led households, female-led households are at a higher risk of housing insecurity.

Indigeneity and Housing Insecurity

Housing insecurity, shaped by class and gender, further varies in terms of being Indigenous or non-Indigenous. In 2016, Indigenous households faced higher housing insecurity rates, at 18% compared to 12% for non-Indigenous. Within the Indigenous populations, there is a significant gap between renters and homeowners. Out of over 118,000 Indigenous households dealing with housing insecurity, more than 93,000 were renters, and over 25,000 were homeowners. The Indigenous housing insecurity rates were 34% for renters and 7% for homeowners (CMHC 2020b). Indigenous renters are nearly five times more likely to face housing insecurity compared to Indigenous homeowners.

Race, Ethnicity, and Housing Insecurity

Race, ethnicity, class, and gender all affect housing insecurity. In 2016, while the national average for housing insecurity was 12.7%, it was significantly higher for certain groups: 32% for West Asian, 30% for Korean, and 24% for Arab households (CMHC 2022). Racialized individuals were two to three times more likely to face housing insecurity than those non-racialized individuals. This gap is especially noticeable in renting, where racialized communities had a 32% rate of housing insecurity compared to 25% for non-racialized communities. Among homeowners, over 12% of racialized households faced housing insecurity, double the rate for non-racialized households (CMHC 2022).[7] Renters are generally more at risk of housing insecurity than homeowners, regardless of race, ethnicity, or gender.

In 2018, 13.5% of Indigenous Peoples in Canada experienced core housing need, compared to 8.8% of non-Indigenous people. Those who experienced core housing need reported poorer health and lower life satisfaction and were more likely to live in overcrowded homes or dwellings requiring major repairs. Additionally, Indigenous households were nearly three times more likely to encounter health-related problems such as mildew, mould, and undrinkable water than their non-Indigenous counterparts (Hahmann and Masoud 2023, 3). These figures underscore the persistent issue of housing insecurity across the country.

According to data from Statistics Canada (2024a, 2–5), 10.1% of households in Canada, or roughly one in ten, experienced core housing need in 2021. Homeowners were less likely (5.3%) than renters (20%) to face housing insecurity, which was highest in major urban centres at 18.4%. Housing insecurity was most severe in Nunavut, where 32.9% of households were affected, compared to just 6% in Québec, the province with the lowest rate. Among those in core housing need, 77.1% faced unaffordable housing, 5.5% lived in inadequate housing, 4.4% were in unsuitable housing, and 13% experienced more than one of these challenges simultaneously. Income primarily shapes housing insecurity.

Women, racialized individuals, and renters are more likely to struggle with insecure housing. However, housing insecurity primarily depends on employment income. In 2019, for visible minority status, households earning less than $32,345 were at higher risk of housing insecurity, while those making over $107,070 per year had no problems with affordability, suitability, or having enough space (Edwards 2019, A1). Housing insecurity is a predominantly class issue. Like poverty and food insecurity, our housing policies must account for class and other sociodemographic factors to address such distinct but interrelated issues. However, although gender, race, ethnicity, and being Indigenous affect housing and health, class is the biggest determinant of housing insecurity. It should be noted that housing insecure people impacted by gender, race, ethnicity, and Indigeneity are most often in the lower class — a double or triple whammy but not separate.

Further Reflection

For almost a century, the Canadian capitalist state has funded the building and maintenance of social housing units through different programs. These programs include public housing, cooperative and non-profit housing, low-rental housing, rent-geared-to-income housing, and rent supplement initiatives. They also encompass broader programs like community development, city improvement, and housing renovation.

Between 1949 and 1985, Canada's governments built approximately 205,000 units through the Public Housing Program. From 1973 to 1979, the Cooperative Housing Program added about 7,700 units, and from 1973 to 1993, the Non-Profit Housing Program created roughly 236,000 units (CMHC 2011, 131–35). These policies provided affordable housing to various groups, including war veterans, older adults, people with disabilities, women, children, Indigenous people, and low-income families. Socialized housing protects these marginalized groups from adverse health effects.

Keynesian policies focused on meeting community needs, such as public housing. Subsequent neoliberal policies, however, prioritize private housing. Ruling governments defunded public housing, which worsened when policymakers terminated federal social housing programs. Remarkably, before these changes, homelessness in Canada was uncommon. While the Keynesian approach provided temporary relief, it does not align well with the capitalist system in the long term as it depends primarily on the balance of power between workers and capitalists and political contestations among various social forces.

Despite having the power to tackle inequalities, the Canadian capitalist state has not done enough. Today, about 68% of houses in the country are privately owned, and 27% are privately managed rentals. Only about 5% are part of the community and public "non-market" sector, where rents are set administratively rather than by the market (Pomeroy 2021, 1). Our housing system depends heavily on private market activities for building, owning, and running homes. The government mainly focuses on generating revenue and only acts on housing needs when there is enough political pressure. Without public demand for change, the government's response is typically inadequate.

Statistics Canada reported that social housing accounted for 894,000 units, or 5.4% of the total housing units available nationwide in 2021. Its distribution varies among provinces and territories. Nunavut has the highest proportion of social housing units, accounting for 84.1% of all housing units in the territory. Newfoundland and Labrador has the lowest proportion of social housing units, with only 3.1% of the total housing in the province (Statistics Canada 2023b, 1). The shortage of socialized housing aggravates housing insecurity, forcing people to cope with high costs in the private market for homeownership or rentals. This condition leaves little money for necessities like food, health services, or education.

Housing insecurity and homelessness are still significant issues, highlighting flaws in government housing programs and the nature of capitalist societies. The main problem is our current economic and political systems, which see housing primarily as something to buy and sell in the market instead of something the state should guarantee for everyone. We have seen progress and setbacks in Canada's housing policies from 1935 to the present. Initially, setting up social housing programs in the mid-twentieth century seemed like a good step. However, subsequent changes in policy, like giving more responsibility to local governments, led to less funding and made it more challenging to provide socialized housing. These policy shifts exacerbated housing and health inequities issues.

Housing activists, community organizations, and intergovernmental organizations, like the UN Committee on Economic, Social, and Cultural Rights, have focused more on Canada's poverty and housing problems. This attention led to new efforts, like the National Housing Strategy Act in 2019. Different governments have tried to address housing concerns while supporting the wealthy and capitalist class. Our housing policies are driven not by government's generosity but by political necessity to calm people's worries and prevent societal upheavals. It is also about the ruling government's legitimacy and survival.

Capitalist ideas and practices emphasize individualism and competition, making it hard for socialized housing programs to work well. This perspective means governments in capitalist societies do not help as many people as much as possible. Our current policies are insufficient to handle the growing need for housing, so we need different plans. These new plans should address the unequal way society is divided by class, which is exacerbated by how capitalism further exploits people based on their race, ethnicity, and gender. Housing struggles mean class struggles and political contestations. Therefore, workers and community groups must work together to challenge the alliance between Big Capital and the government. Community collaboration is crucial for addressing the root causes of housing insecurity and homelessness. Socialized housing, where the state provides housing for all, is vital for ensuring everyone has a good place to live and improving health outcomes.

Notes

1   Monetary policy impacts the economy by adjusting the money supply, interest, and exchange rates. In contrast, fiscal policy relies on changing taxation and government spending to manage economic cycles. The Keynesian approach stresses that state intervention through these macroeconomic policies is crucial for preventing and addressing economic crises and promoting growth. In severe downturns, the state might even need to take control of private property (Wolff and Resnick 2012, 105–132). However, these measures still ignore labour and health exploitation inherent in capitalism.

2   Capitalism has been unstable since its emergence, marked by mutual distrust between workers and employers, leading to strikes and power shifts. Competition among employers lowers wages and sometimes results in monopolies. While unions improve conditions, employer resistance causes labour market fluctuations. Capitalism offers upward mobility but deepens social inequalities. Practices like women and low-wage immigrants demanding higher paid jobs exacerbate conflicts. Economic inequalities trigger varying degrees of government intervention and cycling regulation. These instabilities drive changes, increasing capitalism's volatility (Wolff and Resnick 2012, 310–345). Thus, capitalism's contradictions perpetuate its dynamic and turbulent nature.

3   I use the term "Big Capital" to refer to big businesses and corporations, ultrarich individuals and families, and large private banks, which exert significant influence over government and society.

4   This initiative leveraged the Vancouver Olympics to raise awareness of homelessness. Media engagement by activists sparked public discourse, and the Vancouver mayor's challenge to provincial and federal governments added urgency to the issue. In June 2007, a UN warning about displacements triggered a human rights complaint, followed by a Special Rapporteur's visit in the fall of 2007, resulting in a condemning report on homelessness in Canada. This period also saw the establishment of the Mental Health Commission. These developments, along with the Federation of Canadian Municipalities' call for a national housing strategy, paved the way for the At Home/Chez Soi project (Borras 2022, 64–66). Political struggles significantly influenced housing and health policy.

5   For an in-depth discussion on homelessness-related policy and health inequities in Canada, see Borras, Komakech, and Raphael 2023.

6   Data is available in the tables in CMHC 2020a and 2020b.

7   Please refer to the tables in CMHC 2022.

CHAPTER THREE

Neoliberalism and Canada's Health Care System

The British North America Act of 1867 significantly impacted Canada's health care system, splitting the responsibilities between the federal and provincial governments. The federal government was to be responsible for quarantine and marine hospitals, while the provinces managed other health institutions. From 1897 to 1919, the Department of Agriculture handled federal health matters (Government of Canada 2019), underscoring how health was tied to the economy and food system. After World War I, Canada set up its first Department of Health, which was a major advancement because it showed the government becoming more involved in public health.

Transition from Private to Public Health Care System

Canada's health care system underwent significant changes after World Wars I and II. In the 1920s, Alberta, Manitoba, Saskatchewan, and British Columbia began moving toward a public health care system. These provinces created plans for hospitals run by the local governments and explored health insurance programs. Alberta and British Columbia had implemented health insurance policies by 1936. In the 1940s, we saw the emergence of Keynesianism, the Federal Dominion Council of Health was established, and a federal committee to advise on health insurance was formed (Government of Canada 2019). This action centralized health care policy at the federal level.

Subsequently, in 1947, Saskatchewan introduced a hospital insurance plan for everyone, which sparked changes across Canada. The federal government started the National Health Grants Program the following year, providing money for different health projects (Statistics Canada n.d.).

Then, in 1957, the Hospital Insurance and Diagnostic Services Act created a system where the federal government and provinces shared the cost of hospital insurance. This policy faced opposition from the insurance industry and doctors. However, from 1958 to 1960, most provincial governments followed this care model (Government of Canada 2019). These changes shifted our health care from being primarily privately funded to a system where the government (public) paid, but most services were still private.

Tug of War toward Socialist-Oriented Publicly Funded Universal Health Care

Canada made significant strides in its health care system from the early 1960s to the 1970s. For instance, despite pushback from the Canadian Medical Association, Québec began sharing health care costs with the federal government in 1961. Around the same time, the Royal Commission on Health Services was established. A pivotal moment came in 1962 when Saskatchewan launched public health care and an insurance plan, which led to a twenty-three-day strike by doctors (Government of Canada 2019), backed by pharmaceutical and insurance companies. Workers' unions, farmers' groups, community organizations, and most health care workers supported the fight for universal health care.

During this Keynesian period, intense debates and clashes occurred between those who supported the universal health care system, such as left-leaning parties and social movements, and opponents, such as elite physicians and pro-capitalist parties attached to neoclassical economics. This disagreement led to the Saskatoon Agreement, which supported a fee-for-service payment system (Taylor 2011; TommyDouglas Tube 2012). Rather than transformative politics, this transactional and compromising approach contributed to a weaker form of public health care, which in turn has contributed to the current health care crisis.

In 1963, the Liberal Party secured victory in the federal election, and subsequently, the Royal Commission on Health Services recommended a universal health care program. By 1965, British Columbia had rolled out its medical plan. The year 1966 was crucial, marking the launch of the Canada Assistance Plan and the Medical Care Act, which signalled a transition from private to public health care funding by introducing 50/50 cost-sharing medical insurance plans for provinces and territories (Government of Canada 2019). This policy change towards shared health care financing responsibility grew over the years, with most provincial/territorial governments adopting cost-sharing plans.

There were substantial changes in health care policy from the mid-1970s to the early 1980s. For example, in 1977, the Federal-Provincial Fiscal Arrangements and Established Programs Financing Act shifted funding from shared costs to block grants (Government of Canada 2019). This policy shift gave the provinces and territories more freedom in how health care funds were used. Then, because doctors charged patients extra, the Canadian Labour Congress helped organize the Canadian Health Coalition in 1979 (CHC 2016). This coalition, composed of older adults, women, health care workers, anti-poverty activists, and religious groups, showed how civil society, including the workers' movement, can tackle problems in our health care system.

The political landscape changed again when the Progressive Conservative Party won in 1979, and the Liberal Party returned in 1980. This change led to efforts to make health care standards consistent nationwide and prevent doctors from charging patients extra. In 1981, an agreement was made for hospitals to bill each other for services, with provinces and territories collaborating closely on providing health services. By 1982, the Established Programs Financing was changed to remove a revenue guarantee. The following year, the government created the Federal Task Force on Health Care Resource Allocation, and Newfoundland and Québec mandated commissions to manage their health care resources better and control costs (Government of Canada 2019).

In the mid- to late 1980s, radical changes happened: The 1984 Canada Health Act established important care principles, such as ensuring ease of access to and uniformity of care across provinces and territories. It also guarantees that doctors cannot charge patients extra or ask for user fees (Minister of Justice 2024). Although the Progressive Conservative Party won in 1984 and funds given to provinces were substantially reduced in 1986, all provincial/territorial governments follow the Canada Health Act. Furthermore, Alberta, Nova Scotia, and Ontario conducted in-depth reviews of their care systems, adding to the national conversation about health services. By 1988, all governments except Québec agreed to share physician billing between provinces.

The Continuing Private War against Universal Health Care

In the late 1980s and 1990s, federal transfer payments to provinces and territories were decreased by the Mulroney regime, which aggressively implemented neoliberal policies. Despite deep cuts, provincial inquiries, such as those conducted by British Columbia's Royal Commission (1990–91) and Prince Edward Island's Task Force (1991–92), persisted. Additionally, the Canadian Institute for Health Information was founded to improve health information management and research. The Liberal Party's election in 1993 encouraged further discussions through the National Forum on Health (1994–97) (Government of Canada 2019).

A radical policy shift in 1995 under Finance Minister Paul Martin Jr. combined the Federal Established Programs Financing and Canada Assistance Plan into the Canada Health and Social Transfer, reducing federal health spending from 10.2% of the GDP in 1992 to 9.2% in 1995 (CHC 2016), a massive cut of over $6 billion in one year. From 1985 to 1995, six federal budgets diminished health and social funding by $30 billion, with further cutbacks of $11.2 billion through 1998–99 (Naylor, Boozary, and Adams 2020, E1409).

In 1997, Québec initiated a mandatory pharmacare program, integrating private and public drug coverage (CHC 2016). New Brunswick released its Health Services Review in 1999, the same year governments (excluding Québec) signed the Social Union Framework Agreement to unify social and health care policies. The Northwest Territories also conducted a health care review, reporting in 2000 (Government of Canada 2019).

In the early 2000s, the Ministers' Communiqué on Health agreed upon health goals, and the Canadian Institutes of Health Research was established. Notably, Québec's Commission of Study on Health and Social Services further influenced health care policy (Government of Canada 2019), while Alberta moved towards care privatization, highlighted by Premier Klein's plans for private hospitals and Bill 11. Various provincial bodies also released their health care system assessments, and Canada Health Infoway was launched to modernize the health services.

In 2001, the Kirby Committee began reviewing Canada's health care system, releasing its report in October 2002. Senator Kirby's role as a board member of the for-profit company Extendicare Inc. raised concerns about potential conflicts of interest (CHC, 2016). Concurrently, the Romanow Royal Commission started on April 4, producing its report in November 2002 (Government of Canada 2019). The Romanow Commission suggested health care policy changes, like setting up the Health Council of Canada, ensuring funding lasts a long time, organizing care better, and improving medical tests and training. The commission also recommended that the federal government pay for at least 25% of the provinces' and territories' health care spending (Naylor, Boozary, and Adams 2020, E1409). However, many of these policy ideas did not materialize, showing the differences between research, what is proposed, and what gets done.

In 2003, officials established the Ministers' Accord on Health Care Renewal and the Canadian Patient Safety Institute (Government of Canada 2019), allowing private sector involvement in the health care system. Following the Liberal Party's victory in the federal election, 2004 saw the Canada Health and Social Transfer split into the Canada Health Transfer and Canada Social Transfer, alongside the creation of the Public Health Agency of Canada and the First Ministers' 10-Year Plan to Strengthen Health Care. Ontario also passed the Commitment to the Future of Medicare Act in 2004 (Government of Canada 2019).

Since 2003, provincial and territorial governments have aimed for cash transfers to constitute 25% of total health care spending. The 2004 First Ministers' meeting led to a ten-year accord, a $41.3 billion health care agreement featuring a $35.3 billion boost to the Canada Health Transfer. This increase included immediate one-time surges over two years, a 6% annual growth target, medical equipment allocations, and wait-time reductions (Naylor, Boozary, and Adams 2020, E1409). The Federal Advisor on Wait Times published its concluding report in 2006.

Major changes in health care policy occurred during Harper's regime, from the mid-2000s to the mid-2010s. In 2006, the Senate Committee on Social Affairs, Science, and Technology released the Kirby Report focusing on mental health, while Alberta and British Columbia introduced health care policy guides. In 2007, the Mental Health Commission of Canada and the Canadian Partnership Against Cancer were established (Government of Canada 2019). Additionally, the government started the Patient Wait Times Guarantee initiative.

In 2008, provinces unveiled strategic health plans targeting specific provincial health needs; these included Alberta's Health Action Plan and Vision 2020, Manitoba's Regional Health Authority Report, New Brunswick's Provincial Health Plan 2008–12, and Nova Scotia's Changing Health Care System (Government of Canada 2019). The House of Commons Standing Committee on Health assessed the 2004 Accord's impact on health care progress.

Remarkably, in 2012, federal funding cuts to the Interim Federal Health Programme restricted refugees' access to treatments for chronic health conditions such as angina, diabetes, and hypertension, posing a health services challenge for marginalized groups. In 2013, the government withdrew funding from the Health Council of Canada (CHC 2016), impacting health planning, innovation, and accessibility. The council had played a crucial role in reducing wait times and fostering innovation in the public health care system.

In 2014, the Health Accord ended, which meant federal funding was given to provinces and territories with no strings attached, leading to different levels of public health care coverage. Moreover, funding tied to economic growth meant less money for health services. Consequently, provincial and territorial governments were predicted to be short $43.5 billion in funding by 2024–25 (CHC 2016). During the Harper regime, the state continued the neoliberal austerity policies started by Mulroney, which significantly weakened the health care system by moving from universal care toward privatized care.

Toward Privatized Health Care or Socialized Medicine?

In 2015, Justin Trudeau's government dropped the appeal against a 2014 court ruling that deemed refugee health care benefit cuts unconstitutional. Then, in 2017, federal, provincial, and territorial governments agreed on the Common Statement of Principles on Shared Priorities to enhance community, home care, and mental health services, even though detailed action plans were lacking. The federal government pledged $11 billion over ten years for these priorities, beginning with $150 million in 2017–18 for the opioid crisis. Federal health care spending, initially at 19.6% of provincial/territorial expenditures in 2004–05, rose to 23.2% by 2019–20, with annual adjustments tied to economic growth, ensuring a minimum 3% increase (Marchildon, Allin, and Merkur 2020, 72). However, this budget fell below the proposed 25% federal funding level advocated by Romanow and supported by provincial/territorial governments.

In 2023, Trudeau and the provincial/territorial leaders discussed maintaining the Canada Health Act. The federal government announced an additional health care budget for the provinces and territories over the next decade, totalling $196.1 billion. This budget includes $46.2 billion in new money and an additional $2 billion for Indigenous health care needs. They highlighted four areas they want to focus on: (1) enhancing access to health services for families, especially in rural areas; (2) supporting health care workers and reducing patient backlogs; (3) improving mental health services and aiding people with substance use issues; and (4) modernizing the health care system with better data and digital tools (Prime Minister of Canada 2023). The new health care direction appears promising.

The recent injection of $19.61 billion annually into health care funding is undoubtedly a step in the right direction. However, it is essential to note that this amount does not meet the provinces' request for a yearly $28 billion increase in federal health transfers (Duong 2023, E311). Such an increase would have been pivotal in reverting to a better cost-sharing arrangement, similar to that which existed before the era of intensified neoliberalism.

Projections suggested that total health care expenditure in Canada would reach $344 billion in 2023, an increase of over $9 billion from the previous year. This represents a growth rate of 2.8% in 2023, following a sluggish increase of 1.5% in 2022. (Note: Data for actual expenditure is unavailable at the time of writing.) This minimal increase starkly contrasts with the substantial spikes of 13.2% in 2020 and 7.8% in 2021, primarily driven by the demands of the COVID-19 pandemic. Annual health care spending experienced an average increase of 4.3% per year over the five years leading up to the pandemic (CIHI 2023a). Unfortunately, the additional federal funding does not keep pace with inflation, population growth, and the increasing health care needs of an aging populace.

Hence, asserting that the recent budgetary adjustment will completely rectify the adverse effects of past cuts on Canada's health care system and public health is premature, overly optimistic, and potentially misleading to the public for political purposes. Our health care system has been considerably compromised, as evidenced by factors such as the projected shortage of nurses alone, estimated at 117,600 by 2030 (Scheffler and Arnold 2019, 283–84). We are facing severe shortages of health care workers, and the budget does not provide sufficient assurance that these deficiencies will be adequately addressed.

Overall, the recent health care policy actions of the federal, provincial and territorial governments are largely shaped by lessons learned from dealing with COVID-19 and past budget cuts. By augmenting the health care budget, the government aims to ensure everyone can access health care, improve the quality of care, support health care workers, and leverage technology to improve the system. An underfunded health care system worsens inequalities in care services. Territories and smaller provinces suffer the most because they do not have the financial resources to compensate for the cutbacks. Consequently, the quality of health services varies significantly among the classes in these jurisdictions.

Furthermore, when public funding decreases, there is more pressure to turn to private health services, which increases costs for patients and their families. As a result, lower income families and individuals rarely get the care they need. The existence of private health care creates a system where wealthier individuals receive better care, which goes against Canada's promise of equal health care for all.

The Canada Health Act

The Canada Health Act of 1984 established publicly funded health insurance (Medicare) to ensure accessible health services. The Canada Health Act sets standards for insured and extended health services by provinces and territories. The federal government supports the provinces and territories in maintaining national care standards, while those governments manage and provide health services in line with the Act's guidelines. The Canada Health Act's five principles guarantee that provinces and territories uphold the following care standards to receive total federal funding:

1. *Public Administration.* Non-profit organizations should manage health plans funded by the government and be transparent about their finances. They should be regularly audited to make sure they are operating correctly. Some responsibilities can be awarded to agencies, but the public should oversee them.
2. *Comprehensiveness.* Health plans should cover all essential medical services, including those provided by hospitals, doctors, and dentists. They might also include more services required by provincial or territorial laws.
3. *Universality.* Everyone in the health plan should receive the same benefits, regardless of their social identity. This requirement ensures that everyone can access health services without any unfair treatment.
4. *Portability.* Health plans should allow people to receive care promptly, even if they move or travel. They should facilitate services outside their home area, and payments should match local rates. People waiting for a new plan should still be able to receive care.
5. *Accessibility.* Health plans should allow everyone to use the health care system without incurring excessive costs. Service payments should be fair, based on what the province or territory decides (Minister of Justice 2024, 6–8).

Despite the rules in place, there is still an ongoing conflict between publicly funded and privately funded health care, affecting how Canada's health care system works. Nevertheless, the Canada Health Act still guarantees people health services based on need, not financial capability. These assurances have remained relatively robust for over forty years, even though some aspects have changed because of neoliberal state policies.

Brief Critique of the Canada Health Act

The Canada Health Act has some major issues: (1) it has a lower legal status and limited legal power; (2) most of the money spent on health care comes from the government (public), but a significant portion also comes from private sources;[1] (3) even though the government pays for a lot of it, many health services are provided by private companies; (4) the Act only covers medically necessary services, leaving out essential health care needs like prescription drugs and dental care; (5) different levels of government have different ideas about what health services are necessary, leading to variations in coverage and care; (6) there are disagreements about how health coverage should work when people travel between provinces; and (7) some people who do not have official health care coverage face extra difficulties accessing health services, resulting in long waits for care and out-of-pocket expenses. These problems create inequalities in health and care, showing that changes are needed to ensure everyone gets health services fairly and quickly.

Closing the Gaps

The limitations of the Canada Health Act showcase the necessity for expanding health services. First, the lack of universal pharmacare results in fluctuating provincial/territorial support and private insurance, exacerbating socioeconomic and health disparities. Specifically, 3.6 million individuals faced challenges affording medications, with 700,000 lacking coverage in 2017 (Roh 2019). By 2021, 21% of people in Canada were without prescription insurance, mainly due to low income or unemployment. Inequalities are particularly stark between racialized (29%) and non-racialized persons (14%), immigrants (29%) and non-immigrants (17%), and those over 65 (25%) and aged 25 to 64 (18%). Provincial coverage gaps vary from 26% uninsured in British Columbia to 14% in Nova Scotia (Cortes and Smith 2022, 1–3).

In British Columbia, Prince Edward Island, and Ontario, where more people do not have health insurance, fewer people can get the medication they need. People without insurance are much less likely to take their medication regularly, and many spend out of pocket for it (Cortes and Smith 2022, 7–9). This is a severe situation because Canada's drug prices are among the highest worldwide (Government of Canada 2023). Major policy changes are necessary to guarantee that everyone can get the medication they need, especially people who are struggling financially, racial minorities, immigrants, and older adults in different parts of the country.

On February 29, 2024, the New Democratic Party and Liberal Party introduced a national pharmacare plan called Bill C-64: An Act Respecting Pharmacare. Under this plan, if you have a health card, you will no longer have to pay for diabetes medication or birth control (Parliament of Canada 2024). This move is partly about ensuring everyone can afford the medicine they need, but it is also a strategic political play. With an election on the horizon in 2025, both parties are looking to gain favour with voters by pushing for significant changes in health services.

Second, there are significant gaps in mental health care coverage under the Canada Health Act. Although family doctors and psychiatrists are crucial for mental health care, services such as psychological counselling require private insurance or out-of-pocket payment. Approximately 5.3 million people need mental health support, but only 3 million receive all the care they need, 1.2 million receive partial care, and 1.1 million receive no care at all. A substantial portion of those who need counselling do not receive it (34%), whereas most who need medication do (85%) (Statistics Canada 2019a, 3).

Problems with mental health care affect people based on their income levels, geographical location, and access to regular mental health providers. People with the lowest incomes are more likely not to get the care they need (51%) compared to those with the highest incomes (38%). In Ontario (46%) and British Columbia (51%), many people are not getting the care they need. People without regular mental health care providers are more likely not to get help (60%) than those who have them (41%). Problems getting enough mental health care include (1) not being able to afford it, (2) not knowing where to go for help, (3) not speaking the same language, and (4) trying to manage things on their own (Statistics Canada 2019a, 4–5).

During the COVID-19 pandemic, mental health issues worsened, especially for people without jobs. Racialized minorities and gender-diverse individuals also experienced increased problems. Mental health significantly declined for young people aged 15 to 24 but not for those over 65. Unfortunately, Canada spends less on mental health services compared to other Organisation for Economic Co-operation and Development (OECD) nations, allocating only 7% of the total health expenditure as of 2017 (CIHI 2019, 13). In 2021, Canada allocated 10.6% of its total government health spending to mental health, less than France, Germany, and Norway but higher than some other OECD countries (OECD 2021, 24–25). By improving accessibility to mental health services, we can provide better support for those facing mental health issues.

Third, excluding most dental care services from the Canada Health Act results in significant access gaps. In 2018, 6.8 million individuals avoided dental care due to cost, with females more likely to forgo visits (24.1%) than males (20.6%), and 28.3% of those aged 18–34 cited cost as a barrier. Only 64.6% of people had dental insurance, and 82.5% of those with insurance sought dental care, compared to 60.5% without insurance. Those lacking insurance were more likely to avoid visits due to cost (39.1%) than insured individuals (13.7%). Income level notably influences dental care access, with high-income insured individuals more likely to visit dentists (88.5%) than uninsured low-income individuals (49.6%) (Statistics Canada 2019b, 5).

Our public funding for dental care is insufficient, covering only 6% compared to the OECD average of 31% (Flood et al. 2023, 12). In 2019, we spent $16.4 billion on dental care, but most (94%) was paid privately (Canadian Dental Association 2023). Not being able to access dental care when needed can negatively impact overall health, mental well-being, social life, and job performance (Doucet 2023). Although in 2023 the government promised $13 billion over five years to support uninsured families in getting dental care, experts believe we need a better plan, such as creating a national agency for dental care (Flood et al. 2023, 3). We need a comprehensive plan that includes better financing and a shift in how we think about dental care.

Fourth, long-term care (LTC) homes, such as nursing homes, assist people with physical or medical needs. Nevertheless, there are differences: 46% of these homes are public, and 54% are privately owned, with some being for-profit and others not-for-profit (CIHI 2021). Different parts of the country have different preferences for the ownership of these homes (see Table 3.1). About 11% of our health budget goes to these homes, mostly from public sources (Marchildon, Allin, and Merkur 2020, 61). The Canada Health Act usually does not cover LTC services. However, the government assists with personal care, nursing care, and living costs based on income. Each province or territory decides who gets into these homes, often based on age, memory problems, or ongoing illnesses.

TABLE 3.1 OWNERSHIP OF LONG-TERM CARE HOMES IN CANADA

Province or Territory	Total LTC homes	Public (%)	Private (%)	Private For-Profit (%)	Private Not-For-Profit (%)
Newfoundland	40	98	2	0	2
Prince Edward Island	19	47	53	47	6
Nova Scotia	84	14	86	44	42
New Brunswick	70	0	100	14	86
Québec	440	88	12	n/a	n/a
Ontario	627	16	84	57	27
Manitoba	125	57	43	14	29
Saskatchewan	161	74	26	5	21
Alberta	186	46	54	27	27
British Columbia	308	35	65	37	28
Yukon	4	100	0	0	0
Northwest Territories	9	100	0	0	0
Nunavut	3	100	0	0	0

Note: The author created the table using CIHI 2021 data. "n/a" indicates that data is not available.

Nursing homes' quality of care differs depending on whether for-profit or not-for-profit. Not-for-profit homes usually provide more hands-on care and have better outcomes. During the early pandemic, the proportion of COVID-19 deaths that happened in LTC homes in Canada (81%) was significantly higher than the OECD average (38%) (CIHI 2020a, 2). Residents in government-run and not-for-profit homes had fewer infections and deaths than those in for-profit homes (Oved et al. 2020). These inequalities highlight problems such as staffing shortages and inadequate infection prevention measures in for-profit nursing homes (Borras 2023, 140).

Health inequalities in long-term care demonstrate how neoliberal policies have increasingly privatized LTC, leading to budget cuts and lower-quality care and working conditions. The pandemic further revealed the inner workings of LTC. It showed how funding, different kinds of LTC homes, rules, and government policies affect LTC practices. This scenario has prompted us to ask important questions and consider making bold changes to LTC operations.

Fifth, in 2021, about 6% of Canada's households (roughly 921,700) received formal home care services, while nearly half of those needing home care (419,800) did not receive any. Among those receiving home care, 48% received only medical services, 32% received help with daily tasks, and 20% received both. In regions with more elderly residents, home care usage was higher (10%), whereas low-income suburban areas had lower usage (8%) and higher unmet needs (4%) compared to high-income regions (2%). Factors such as being a single parent, education, home ownership, income, and employment impact how people utilize home care, particularly in low-income areas (Statistics Canada 2022a, 1). Unmet home care needs, especially in low-income suburban regions, highlight the need for state intervention.

Last but not least, Canada's health care system grapples with prolonged wait times, notably for specialist services, elective surgeries, and diagnostics. Emergency department waits in urban centres exceed those in many countries, with 29% of patients enduring waits over four hours (Marchildon, Allin, and Merkur 2020, 142). Despite government efforts to alleviate wait times since the early 2000s, outcomes have been mixed. For example, benchmarks for sight restoration and joint replacements frequently go unmet, though cancer radiation therapy targets are often achieved. While the median wait for cataract surgery falls below the OECD average, it still exceeds that of some nations. Wait times for hip and knee replacements surpass the OECD average. Long-term care homes also face concerns about wait times. Median wait times for admission have surged, leaving thousands on waitlists (Marchildon, Allin, and Merkur 2020, 142–44).

The escalating demand for home care due to an aging population and unmet needs among younger individuals with chronic conditions further compound waiting issues (Marchildon, Allin, and Merkur 2020). The shortage of health workers contributes to long wait times; for example, some patients cannot get care because doctors are not taking new patients due to overcapacity. Additionally, waiting to see a doctor is getting longer because more people need care. Therefore, we must find ways to recruit and retain more health care workers.

Under the Canada Health Act we are missing essential services like prescription drugs, mental health care, dental care, long-term care, and home care, and we need to address this quickly. While some people advocate for private health services, we need to focus on improving our public care system. We must expand our health care system and change some rules to handle this.

Health Care Policies in the Neoliberal Era

Canada's health care system has undergone significant changes over the years. Notably, in the neoliberal era, we have been spending less on public health care. Federal spending cuts have led to the closure of smaller hospitals and increased workloads for larger ones, resulting in fewer available hospital beds. This shortage has affected Canada's standing in international comparisons of hospital beds, medical imaging, and the adoption of new health care technologies (Marchildon, Allin, and Merkur 2020). The COVID-19 pandemic starkly revealed the detrimental impact of neoliberal policies, forcing hospitals to use temporary facilities to care for patients.

Ontario's Tales of Cuts and Privatization

Ontario's extensive austerity measures exemplify neoliberalism. For instance, the Ford government aggressively implemented health care policies favouring private insurance by altering the Ontario Health Insurance Plan, cutting overdose prevention funding and reducing the Health System Research Fund by $53 million. Additionally, budget cuts led to over 120 job losses across various positions at Health Sciences North in Sudbury. Despite some policy reversals following public protests, significant cuts persisted (OHC 2019, 1–7). More than 1,200 emergency departments and local hospital services were shut down between June 2023 and May 2024 (OHC 2024).

Even before Bill 60, there were attempts to privatize parts of health services, such as lab tests and patient transportation. The Your Health Act (Legislative Assembly of Ontario 2023) further privatized the health care system by allowing the government to appoint "Director/s" — individuals or corporations outside the Ministry of Health. It grants these "Director/s" the power to open private health clinics, transfer licences, and determine the availability and location of services (OHC 2023). This radical shift toward privatized health care makes understanding the system and identifying accountability difficult. It sustains disparities in health services since private companies primarily focus on profit rather than serving people and communities.

Health Workforce Shortages

Neoliberalism's effects on Canada's health care workforce have been profound. In 2021, the number of health care professionals increased: licensed physicians by 2.0%, regulated nurses by 2.4%, and pharmacists by 3.6%. However, the growth rate of family physicians slowed significantly, from

3.4% annually between 2012 and 2014 to just 1.3% between 2019 and 2021. While there are 94,000 physicians, only 8% serve in rural areas, underscoring a stark urban-rural divide in physician distribution. Rural regions, mainly reliant on visiting physicians, faced challenges, with nearly half of Nunavut's family physicians in 2020–21 being non-local (CIHI 2022a, 4).[2] This discrepancy highlights state policy biases towards urban centres.

There are about 459,000 nurses in Canada. This workforce includes 312,400 registered nurses, 132,900 practical nurses, 7,400 nurse practitioners, and 6,350 psychiatric nurses. The Northwest Territories, Nunavut, and Yukon have more nurse practitioners per capita, partly due to a shortage of doctors (CIHI 2022a, 4). Moreover, nurse practitioners are paid significantly less than physicians, allowing the capitalist state to cut costs by lowering care standards. Budget cuts and the effects of colonialism and institutional racism exacerbate this problem in these territories.

While the number of nurses grows, fewer nurses work directly with patients in long-term care and hospitals due to staff shortages, increased workloads, stress, and burnout. Instead, more nurses work for community health agencies and other settings/employers, such as private nursing agencies and self-employment (CIHI 2024, 3). This changing scene shows nurses seeking better pay in non-traditional settings. This trend of nurses moving to private nursing agencies, often paid for by the government but focused on profit-making, illustrates how the government's focus on privatization can affect job security and the quality of patient care. For-profit care agencies are a significant threat to publicly funded health care systems.

During the COVID-19 pandemic, personal support workers in LTC were highly essential. However, 83% faced emotional stress and financial difficulties (Statistics Canada 2022b, 1). It is vital to support personal support workers to help prevent further erosion of our health care system. Furthermore, 96% of people receiving long-term home care rely on unpaid caregivers, who provide approximately 38 hours of care per week. More than a third of these caregivers experience stress, making it hard to continue providing care (CIHI 2020b). We need to support these informal caregivers as they, too, are essential health care workers.

Extended Hours of Work

In 2020–21, the hospital sector saw a 15% surge in overtime (OT) hours among health care workers, totalling over 18 million hours, equivalent to the workload of over 9,000 full-time employees. Nursing staff accounted for approximately 9.8 million OT hours, equivalent to over 5,000 full-time roles. Additionally, there was a 5.5% rise in reliance on agency staff, amounting to 13.7 million hours (CIHI 2022b, 6). These elevated OT rates signify mounting pressures on staff and strain on the health care system's capacity. However, resorting to private agency staff, which aligns with neoliberal policies that favour private resources, often results in fragmented care and serves as a short-term fix for staffing shortages.

Heavy Workload and Health

Health care workers have worked long hours during the pandemic, and most feel stressed (86.5%). They also have more work to do, with 75% saying their workload increased. Nurses are more stressed (92%) than doctors (83.7%), personal support workers (83%), and other health care workers (83%) (Statistics Canada 2022b, 1). This demanding work situation has led many nurses to consider quitting. Thus, workers' groups must advocate for better pay, shorter hours, and improved working conditions. This fight must extend beyond changes within the capitalist system to ensure workers are safe and patients receive excellent care.

The Case of Ontario

Ontario is facing a massive problem due to a need for more health care workers. In 2022, 14,575 nursing jobs and 12,300 personal support worker jobs were vacant. Moreover, nurses in Ontario earn less than their counterparts in other provinces. Personal support workers make 1.3% less than the national average, which is a major concern because living costs in Ontario are higher. Ontario will need even more nurses and personal support workers in the next few years to meet government plans, such as creating more hospital and long-term care beds and providing more home care (FAO 2023, 30–41). However, unions and health advocacy groups have not pushed hard enough to break the alliance between large businesses and the state, further weakening the publicly funded health care system.

Further Reflection

Canada's health care policies, like housing policies, are influenced by power struggles among state players, businesses, and people's movements. The ruling government prioritizes making money, which aligns with the interests of big companies. Nevertheless, it must also listen to what the public wants, especially when the people apply significant pressure. Thus, the government tries to make rules that satisfy both the public and businesses, allowing companies to be part of public sectors like health care.

The incessant struggles among social forces shape state policies, which, in turn, influence population health outcomes.

Our health care policies can be divided into four distinct periods of struggles: transition from private to public health care system (1867–1962), tug of war toward socialist-oriented publicly funded universal health care (1962–84), continuing private war against universal health care (1984–2015), and toward privatized health care or socialized medicine? (2015–present). These periods are marked by ongoing economic and political struggles among classes and groups divided into two irreconcilable factions: pro-capitalist-oriented private health care and pro-socialist-oriented public health care.

The Canada Health Act, though limited in scope, emerged as a result of public health care advocates countering private health care interests. Despite the Act's intention to provide universal health services, the ruling government's adherence to the capitalist system and support for Big Capital has hindered this goal. The Canada Health Act embodies elements of socialist-oriented ideals and aspirations for health equity, but it remains a hybrid of public and private provisioning, resulting in a weaker health care system. There is an ongoing conflict between proponents of public health care and supporters of private health care. Ultimately, the organized classes and groups, supported by the majority of the population, will determine the future direction of Canada's health care system.

Our health care system showed weaknesses both before and during the COVID-19 pandemic. Profit-centred agendas have further eroded the Canada Health Act's core principles. Therefore, shifting away from neoliberalism toward a new societal system where health care is seen as a fundamental human need and a universal right, not a profit-driven commodity, is crucial. This alternative system requires a new societal framework built on solidarity, fairness, and humanity, prioritizing health over financial and personal gain.

Notes

1. Health care spending in Canada has remained consistent over the years. From the early 2000s to 2023, the public sector covered about 70% of total health care expenditure, while the private sector covered about 30% (CIHI 2023b).
2. To access tables and graphs, refer to CIHI (2022c).

CHAPTER FOUR

Political Power and Policy Advocacy

Power dynamics among governments, big businesses, and civil society groups shape health policy. Examples from the United States, United Kingdom, Australia, and Canada demonstrate how these competing interest groups struggle to influence state policy in their favour. Policy changes can vary from minor adjustments to major overhauls, depending on the balance of power among these social forces. The elites, such as capitalists and wealthy people, wield more influence than the masses, including workers and people living in poverty, in shaping state policies to their advantage. Addressing this power imbalance is crucial to preventing, reducing, and eradicating health inequities.

Health Politics

Politics is the study of influence and those who wield it. Typically, the elites — those with more wealth and power — benefit the most from societal resources, including positions of power, wealth, income, and health protection, while the masses receive less. Since politics determines "who gets what, when, how" (Lasswell 1958), politics is a battleground where competing policy actors contend for societal resources. Politics, while being a source of inequities in health and health care, can also be a means to address such inequities.

Health politics explores how theories, processes, and political factors influence decisions made by governing bodies, which in turn affect health outcomes. Health is political in several ways: (1) health is treated as a commodity; (2) political decisions and interventions affect the social determinants of health; (3) people's health is considered both a right and a part of citizenship; and (4) power is used to control health within economic and political systems (Bambra, Fox, and Scott-Samuel 2005, 187).

Health inequities are not just medical issues; they are socioeconomic and political problems that require social activism and political action, such as advocating for state policies that promote fairness in health access and outcomes. Achieving health equity necessitates political struggle.

Policy is a carefully formulated plan that decision makers choose to solve a problem by deciding how to use the available resources. There are two kinds of policy: private (like rules in a company) and public (like rules made by the government). Public policy deals with significant issues, like health inequities, that affect everyone. It is about what the government does or does not do to handle these problems (Dye 2017; Jones 1984; Walt 1994). Health inequities are political issues, and the state is a crucial political arena for reducing health inequities. Notably, the state is responsible for distributing the social determinants of health through public policies. These policies can either make things fairer, make them worse, or make it hard to solve them.

Health policy is a component of public policy aimed at improving health outcomes and promoting equity by addressing various factors, including the social determinants of health. It involves creating, legislating, and implementing policies and programs that influence population health. Within this broader context, *health care policy* specifically targets the financing, delivery, and organization of health care systems and services, ensuring that these systems are structured to effectively meet the population's health care needs.

Policy change means adjusting the current policies or a group of related policies. These changes can happen quickly (radical) or slowly (incremental). Knowing how policies change helps us understand how they are created and enforced, identify what prevents us from addressing health inequities with policies, and find ways to overcome these obstacles (Bryant and Raphael 2016). Understanding public policy means understanding politics. Politics and policy involve how individuals and groups participate in and are represented in state decision-making processes that impact societal life.

Political Participation and Representation

In today's representative democracies and parliamentary systems, many believe that democracy is the best way to govern. Proponents argue that everyone has a fair chance to influence government decisions, especially when addressing social and health problems (Dahl 1961, 1–10). However, the question of who controls power in a democracy within a capitalist system remains unclear. Although democracy ideally ensures that everyone has an equal say, the reality in a capitalist context is that different people and groups possess varying levels of power and influence over state decisions. We must continually assess the integrity of our democratic ideals and practices. There is a prevailing idea that the policymaking process primarily unfolds within the executive, legislative, and judicial branches of the government. Many assume that every person, group, or organization has an equal chance to pursue their policy goals and objectives (Dahl 1984, 1–10), such as reducing health inequities. Under polyarchy — governance by many — the state is perceived as an unbiased intermediary in societal and public health matters (Bryant 2016, 58–60). As a result, most people who support specific policies believe they can make health better by discussing issues, gathering evidence, suggesting ideas, and pushing for policy changes that government officials will consider. However, although these people see the state as neutral when making policies, we must investigate whether everyone has an equal chance of influencing such policies. Considering the state and its institutions as impartial regarding health policies is overly idealistic.

In liberal democracies like Canada, power centres are assumed to be dispersed across society. Proponents of this view think consensus-based politics mirror the diverse interests of different groups striving for policy shifts and social transformations (Mudde and Kaltwasser 2017, 7–8). Some posit that, given that non-state actors' influence on public policy aligns with their unique needs, power is not centralized in the hands of the strongest competitor. Others assert that since policymaking is consistent with the pressures exerted by multiple stakeholders, health "policy does not move in leaps and bounds." This approach, dubbed "incrementalism" or "muddling through," entails making small, step-by-step political changes to tackle social issues (Lindblom 1959, 84–86). Although many political actors advocate for an incremental approach in policymaking, we must evaluate its efficacy in addressing deeply rooted health inequities.

Unequal Power and Politics

In public policymaking, a small group of rich and powerful people known as the "power elite" has significant control and influence over state policies. They oversee major institutions, such as industries, the government, and the military, and their decisions significantly impact society, both in America and worldwide (Mills 1956, 17). In the UK, the elite "capitalist executive" is primarily responsible for creating and perpetuating unfair differences in health based on class, gender, and race (Scambler 2019, 2).

In Canada, influential business leaders work to formulate state policies that help them accumulate more profit and capital. This power elite has a louder voice through business associations (e.g., Business Council of Canada), think tanks (e.g., Fraser Institute), citizen groups (e.g., Canadian Taxpayers Federation), and lobbying firms (e.g., StrategyCorp) (Langille 2016, 476). Their political actions raise questions about whether their priority is making money for themselves or ensuring the well-being of the general population.

Around the world, Big Capital has great power and influence over state policies that affect how healthy people are. Rich people and big companies control employment, housing, food, and health care policies more than regular working people. Although ruling governments claim they decide independently, their policies benefit big corporations more than they do the workers and communities. The state primarily listens to wealthy capitalists, except in rare cases when public pressure forces it to make decisions against corporate interests. These changes are usually temporary. Neoliberalism has weakened our social programs like public housing and health care. Thus, it is important not to see the state as neutral regarding society and public health matters, for it is not.

Indeed, "market systems imprison policy. Those of us who live in those market-oriented systems that are called liberal democratic exercise significantly less control over policy than we have thought. And we are also less free than we may have thought" (Lindblom 1982, 336). Big Capital's dominant role in shaping public policy and people's lives challenges the notion of a state's impartiality and autonomy. This dynamic raises concerns about actual democratic control and the genuine independence of groups and individuals within capitalist societies.

A vast power gap between classes and groups leads to *corporatism*, where a few big corporations control specific industries (Cawson 1978, 187), such as housing and health care. This setup, called an oligopoly, demonstrates how elite groups influence societal rules. Big companies often shape health policies to their benefit, overshadowing the interests and views of workers and health advocates. Oligarchy highlights the dangers of a small group of powerful people having too much control over societal life. Their political influence undermines the idea that everyone should be equally listened to in societal and public health affairs. Despite claims that ordinary people have a voice, the overwhelming power of the elites in health policies reveals a big gap. Addressing these power imbalances is vital to establishing genuinely democratic societies.

Policy Change Approaches

Power struggles and political battles shape the formation and implementation of state policies. Renowned political scientist John Kingdon (1984/2014) argues that policymaking processes involve three main streams: identifying problems, developing policies, and dealing with politics. These streams influence which social issues get attention and which solutions are considered. It is essential to grasp these three policy components and how they interact in public policymaking. This understanding is vital for anyone trying to influence state policies to promote health equity.

The *identifying problems* stream concerns how policymakers and others identify issues like health inequities. They do this by looking at death rates and health problems or by listening to what people say. They also compare these issues to their beliefs or what is happening elsewhere. Policymakers' perceptions of a problem are fundamental. For example, if they see the struggles of people with disabilities as a matter of civil rights instead of just transportation issues, it can influence their proposed solutions (Kingdon 1984/2014). Thus, it is crucial for people who want to change policies to think carefully about how they frame the problems.

In the *developing policies* stream, groups of policy experts such as government officials, academics, and advocacy organizations present their ideas for new policies. It is like a big mixing pot of ideas. These policy proposals can be rejected, changed, or accepted. For a state policy to be implemented, many factors need to come together: what most people in the country think, the predominant values of a society, what the government is focusing on, how practical the policy is, and how much support or opposition it gets from different groups (Kingdon 1984/2014). Making good health policies is not just about having expertise but also about understanding how external factors, like economics, politics, cultures, and institutions, will affect it.

The *dealing with politics* stream is all about how politics affects public policy. It considers changes in public opinion, what interest groups are doing, who wins elections, and who is in charge. These political events affect the selection of social and health issues for consideration and the endorsement of solutions. Politics is about finding agreements, making deals, and teaming up with others, but it is also unpredictable. Even if policymakers plan well or know what problems need fixing, sudden political changes can completely alter the order of things (Kingdon 1984/2014).

Formulating state policies is not just about solving problems logically. It is also about dealing with the unpredictability of politics.

The streams of identifying problems, developing policies, and dealing with politics usually work separately. Sometimes, they come together, creating *policy windows*, or short opportunities to act (Kingdon 1984/2014). These windows mainly open for two reasons: (1) when a problem becomes a crisis or (2) when a significant political change occurs. At these crucial times, *policy entrepreneurs* step in. They are policy advocates ready to push for specific ideas and who have the evidence and support to back them up. Such change makers prepare and tie their solutions to what is going on politically to make the most of these opening moments (Kingdon 1984/2014). When problems, policies, and politics align, it creates chances for big policy changes. Thus, health policy advocates must be prepared and strategic.

Illustrative Cases

The following examples shows how problems, policies, and politics converged to create (or not create) meaningful health policy change. In the early 1970s, health care costs skyrocketed in the US. At the same time, Senator Edward Kennedy had influence on health policy, which made the Nixon administration nervous because they saw him as a potential opponent in the following election. This political tension made the Nixon team more open to new health policy ideas. However, they faced a challenge as they needed to fit these new policies with the Republican Party's values of limited government role and cost efficiency. That is where Paul Ellwood, a health policy expert, came in. He suggested the idea of health maintenance organizations. When the problems of rising health care costs, political pressure, and Ellwood's policy proposal came together, it created a chance for policy change. Eventually, this led to the Health Maintenance Organization Act of 1973, which expanded health coverage and benefits in the US (Kingdon 1984/2014).

Kingdon's policy change framework, often used by researchers and policy advocates, helps us figure out why social and health inequities exist and how to address them. However, while this model is helpful, it is not sufficient. Responding to the unfair health differences in capitalist countries requires radical changes to the system. Predating Kingdon's policy change approach, the UK's Black Report in 1980 called for a more democratic and unified approach — engaging government representative bodies, employers, and civil society to reduce health inequities. The

Black Report proposed thirty-seven policies focused on information and research, social support, and a strategy beyond the health care system (see Black et al. 1992). However, the UK Conservative government shut the policy window to research-based evidence and policy ideas that might have tackled health inequities between the 1980s and 1990s (Exworthy 2002). These periods saw the intensification of neoliberalism worldwide. When the subsequent Labour government took charge, it targeted health inequities following recommendations in Acheson's *Independent Inquiry into Inequalities in Health*, which made thirty-nine policy proposals to improve areas like employment, poverty, housing, education, and transportation (Acheson 1998). Acheson's report argued that if people and communities keep pushing and changing how things are run, they can improve health policy.

Some researchers connected Kingdon's policy change model with the joined-up government approach. Instead of examining how different levels of government work together (horizontal connections), they studied how local actions fit with the central government's policy goals (vertical interactions). They found that while reducing socioeconomic and health inequities is a big priority at both local and national levels, the following obstacles exist: (1) people working on the policy do not collaborate well; (2) government agencies do not coordinate properly; (3) central government does not evaluate local plans sufficiently; and (4) there are conflicting priorities in policies. Thus, it is essential to keep the policy windows open for change nationally and locally if we want health policies to work in the long run (Exworthy, Berney, and Powell 2002, 81–93), as further evidence suggests below.

In Australia, between 1985 and 2011, few policies addressed the unfair distribution of the social determinants of health. Several reasons caused this lack of progress: First, while health ministers knew about health inequities, they primarily focused on health services. Occasionally, they did address the social determinants of health, such as with the Social Health Strategy and Indigenous housing reforms in remote areas. Second, tackling complex problems like the social determinants of health went against the usual way of making policies, which seeks quick fixes to problems like unequal health care access. Third, the prevailing political ideas favoured individualism, seeing health inequities primarily as a result of personal choices or behaviours rather than broader social factors. Fourth, doctors and other medical professionals predominantly shape health policies, and they focused more on acute care services, which the media and public supported. They also preferred solutions like lifestyle changes, which the politicians readily accepted. Fifth, discussions about the social determinants of health and health inequities faded from policy talks. Lastly, neoliberalism shifted focus away from policies that would redistribute societal resources to help more people and communities (Baum et al. 2013, 140–45). In the end, although people knew about persistent health inequities, significant policy changes that could have effectively addressed such inequities faced barriers from economic, political, cultural, and institutional systems that maintain the capitalist ways of thinking and doing things.

The At Home/Chez Soi project in Canada from 2008 to 2013 followed Kingdon's policy change approach. This project showed that policy-making is not straightforward nor logical; it is messy and hard to predict. In this project, former Senator Kirby acted as a policy entrepreneur to help homeless people with mental health issues (Macnaughton, Nelson, and Goering 2013, 102–06). However, the catch is that although the Conservative government benefited politically from this project, they did not invest much in social housing. As a result, homelessness remains a big problem in the country (Borras 2022, 64–66). While Kirby's model offers ideas for making changes in health policies, in the real world, policymaking processes depend on many factors, and outcomes vary greatly.

Policy windows can come and go quickly. So, some researchers and academics suggest that a good strategy to turn research on health inequities into actual policies is to present substantial evidence and solutions to policymakers at the right time (e.g., see Whitehead, Petticrew and Graham 2004, 818). However, it is tricky because policy windows related to the social determinants of health do not open often, and when they do, governmental departments and policymakers want to fit the research and plans into their political agenda (Carey and Crammond 2015, 138–40). This situation is challenging because the policy ideas of scholars, advocates, and activists might not match what those in charge want to do.

Achieving radical policy change is an uphill task when policy windows remain closed. The question emerges: how can we keep these policy windows open to address health inequities effectively? Some propose introducing evidence-backed policy measures, monitoring progress, and promoting interdepartmental collaboration among government agencies (e.g., Exworthy, Blane, and Marmot 2003, 1916–19). However, as we have shown, while structured methods sound promising, their impact on driving meaningful change for health equity is limited. Consequently, others advocate for dual-directional pressure, from the top (the state and its mechanisms) and the bottom (civil society groups), to address health inequities (e.g., Baum 2007, 94). For some, opening policy windows for health equity requires *political will* (e.g., Baum et al. 2020, 11).

Creating equitable health policies goes beyond relying solely on research-informed ideas and evidence. Enacting significant changes requires collaboration from various levels of government and grassroots movements. It involves diverse tactics and strategies to open up opportunities for policy change, such as combining bottom-up and top-down pressures. Therefore, to combat health inequities, we must unite civil society groups and involve the public in challenging the influence of big corporations on health policies. This sustained pressure from below can compel the state and its apparatuses to make better decisions for all. Pressure from the grassroots can weaken the strong bond between government policymakers and big businesses, paving the way to health equity. Importantly, such pressure must be maintained even when desirable policies are enacted in response. Thinking and acting as if policies achieved are sacrosanct has often led to their reversal.

Unequal Resources, Unequal Policy Influence

The biggest challenge in tackling health inequities is that advocacy and lobby groups do not have the same resources: some are abundant, others scarce. During my interviews with leading Canadian policy academics, advocates, and activists, I asked them if all these groups had an equal chance to change public policy; most said, "No." They all agreed that groups with more money and power have more influence over state policies, including policies shaping the distribution of the social determinants of health. Unequal resources lead to unequal influence on policy decisions about health.

We must ensure that decision making is fair and inclusive at work, in our communities, and in governments. People participate in health politics mainly because of their needs and interests, leading to significant differences in who gets heard and who does not. Political economy professor Greg Albo pointed out that addressing these inequities is crucial for ensuring that policy advocates have a fair chance and access to power and opportunities:

> So, you then break down that unequal structure representation in terms of material interests; that is, who has the wealth, who dominates access, who controls the parties, et cetera. And then, the unequal structure of representation in dealing with the various forms of social inequalities, that is, the social inequalities of class and the social inequalities that come along with gender or racial differentiations in societies in Canada. This is also of national differentiations for First Nations and Indigenous peoples. Historically, a strong unequal representation for the Québécois in the Canadian state ... that's equalized a fair bit over time. But, there are still historical remnants of the unequal representation of the French in the Canadian state structure. (The quotes in this section are from interviews I conducted for my doctoral dissertation, see Borras 2022)

It is essential to close the gap between what we aspire to in equal representation and what actually happens. When people do not have equal access to money, cultural resources, and power, they do not have an equal say in state policy decisions that shape society and health. If individuals and groups have fewer resources, it is harder for them to influence public policy decisions that affect everyone's lives. Another interviewee, a health economist, stated:

> Certainly, there's power and influence differences in different stakeholder groups. So, no, they don't have an equal chance to influence policy ... Certain groups have more clout in the system than others for a variety of reasons. People who are marginalized often have the littlest say: poor people, recent immigrants, people with low educational attainment, little human capital, there's not much wealth. They get very marginalized, and they don't have as much of a say in how their society gets shaped. — Anonymous

People with abundant financial resources have more control over politics, leaving out marginalized groups, who often do not have a voice in government decisions concerning access to health necessities. Indigenous communities are a clear example of this.

> In Northern Ontario, First Nation, for example, that has no clean water, that does not even have basic safe housing

that is healthy for people to live in. For them to get access to government ... they would need money to travel. They would need support to create submissions. They would need not just have a call out for hearings ... They would need to be invited. People would need to go to them and seek out their opinions, to research the conditions ... There has to be extra support: a kind of affirmative action to ensure that marginalized voices that represent those communities that have faced severe discrimination and severe inequality and inequities couldn't possibly even participate. — Natalie Mehra, executive director at the Ontario Health Coalition

Marginalized groups have a hard time making their voices heard in policymaking because of deep-rooted systemic obstacles, lack of connections, and social exclusion. On the other hand, professionals with university degrees and similar socioeconomic statuses mainly control the rules and plans for health services. As a result, these elites ignore the different needs of various communities. A physician interviewee stated:

The decisions that are being made in the halls of power are made by folks of a certain group of society. It's a very homogeneous group ... people who have gone to university, who often have professional roles, and who are making these decisions, and relate to others who are the same economic and social background. I see this a lot in health policy where it strikes me how often, and I count myself among these very privileged people ... when I go to meetings with government, how often we all know each other ... there's a social connection between ... these elites who are involved with the discussion. I don't know if it applies in other sectors, but I suspect it does. But certainly, in health policy, there's a very small circle of people who are all personal connections of one another, colleagues, collaborators, even family, friends, and sometimes even people who have married one other because they find themselves in the same circles, but who are also part of that.

The people at the top who make policies keep power to themselves, meaning less powerful groups do not get to influence health policy.

Our health policies do not consider what rank-and-file workers and ordinary people think. Unfortunately, even when researchers and health policy experts ask for opinions from the community, they do not talk about how the capitalist system creates and maintains inequities. The physician added:

> It's interesting that you worked as a PSW [personal support worker]. This is actually an area of work that we're doing now. PSWs, there's something like a hundred thousand in Ontario. It's a huge group. But how often have we ever heard a PSW on the radio talking about their perspective on the health care system? How often do we hear nurses or others involved in health care? It's almost really kind of this certain small group of academics of health policy, so-called experts, and physicians often who are very much shaping that discussion.

Listening only to academics and doctors — most of them have not experienced poverty and are detached from realities on the ground — gives us a limited view of health and health care. We need to hear from all health care workers to see the whole picture. Valuing the experiences of frontline workers is crucial for a better understanding of health policy. Scholars, advocates, and activists should start from the bottom, get support from regular people, and challenge the powerful groups that control state decisions and maintain the status quo.

An unequal distribution of resources like power, wealth, and social connections in policy advocacy makes the game one-sided. For instance, certain housing advocacy groups obtain more money from the government than others. These well-funded groups, many of which have support through the Social Sciences and Humanities Research Council, are reluctant to criticize the status quo and do not push hard to make radical changes to address inequities. Among my interviewees, nurse activist Cathy Crowe[1] explained:

> Nearly all people in academic institutions and national housing organizations receive funding from the federal government through what you call SSHRC grants ... How can they critique? We've had Housing First going on since the early 2000s. And it's only now that a few of them ... with careful wording, begin to say, we have to have a national

housing program. They received so much money, and they are in such positions of privilege with six-figure salaries ... The Toronto Alliance to End Homelessness has the ear of the government ... They receive funding from wherever ... They have a corporate-style executive director position. And then you have the Shelter and Housing Justice Network. We do not have one dollar. And then you have the Ontario Coalition Against Poverty ... They have a few dollars, very few. But we are the voice. We, two groups, are the voices of people with massive experience from the faith sector, social work, nursing, drop-in sector, and shelter. Some of the people have been doing it, like me, for over 30 years. And do we have the ear of the government? Right now, we do not feel the support of one single city councillor for our work. I mean, it comes in waves.

That some advocacy groups have more resources than others prevents critical perspectives from being heard in policies about housing and health. To really make a difference, we should support local groups that directly work with people experiencing homelessness or struggling with unstable housing. We must question who is benefiting from the fact that widespread housing insecurity and homelessness persist. Many government-funded groups and experts talk about homelessness and housing insecurity, but they rarely blame the capitalist system or suggest abolishing the private property system that shapes housing policy. This neglect is concerning because housing insecurity caused by the free-market system leads to homelessness. It is vital to address this research gap.

In the health care sector, trade unions have the power to shape health policies, but their influence often depends on the government in charge. So far, they have only made minor improvements to existing policies. Strengthening workers' power beyond trade unionism is crucial to achieving health for all. Sharleen Stewart, president of the Service Employees International Union Healthcare, stated:

> It depends greatly on what party is in power as well. I'm really hoping to be able to change some policies for long-term care after coming out of this pandemic. But it's been a challenge and a struggle. We've been able to move in small steps. We have a whole lot more to do and a lot more successful outcomes. We were able to move some of

it, but again, it's not equitable compared to other stronger, more powerful lobbying groups that have a lot of money to influence the government to make the decisions.

Workers and labour movements influence what the government does. Still, it depends on the politics and their power compared to wealthy lobbying groups, especially those supporting Big Capital. Powerful interest groups mainly shape the state's health policies. Big pharmaceutical companies and rich investors who donate money to political campaigns have more policy influence than health care unions, groups for older adults, and health coalitions. Michael Hurley, president of the Ontario Council of Hospital Unions, a division of the Canadian Union of Public Employees, had this to say:

> We don't have the same level of influence if you look at the unions in Ontario in the health care sector and the health coalition, for example. As advocates, some seniors' organizations for improvements to health care they're set off against powerful interests, like the pharmacological companies and the long-term care industry private sector interests. Those companies offer jobs and directorships to politicians and senior bureaucrats. They bankroll campaigns. They are political donors. They employ many people. They're very powerful interests, and they are more influential with a government like this one and probably with a government like the last one.

As big corporations become more involved in non-profit organizations and funding for advocacy groups pushing for societal change decreases, the existing gaps in health policy widen even more. Natalie Mehra further commented:

> In Canada, there has been a very significant change over the last generation in terms of advocacy from non-profit organizations and funding those organizations to support social change. And that has made a huge difference. The non-profit sector has become more corporatized, with corporations on their boards of directors … There's been a sort of neoliberalization of civil society organizations. There have also been very dramatic cuts to government funding. Today, there's almost no funding at all available for advocacy organizations or groups that advocate. The

right-wing groups have gotten around this, but the progressive groups have not been able to.

Some civil society groups have shifted focus to align more with corporate interests and neoliberal ideas. At the same time, government funding for groups trying to make society fairer has diminished, making advocacy efforts more challenging for those groups. To address these issues, we must confront corporate power and influence in grassroots organizations and ensure that advocacy groups have adequate resources from various supporters.

Further Reflection

My findings contradict the claims that health inequities persist mainly due to employment and income inequalities and the limited range and execution of evidence-based policies (e.g., see Mackenbach 2011). They also deviate from claims that the failure to decrease health inequities results from deep-rooted policy paradigms and institutionalized ideas that block research-driven policy proposals (e.g., see Smith 2007, 2013a, 2013b, 2014). Instead, the results of my study support the view that political ideologies aligned with capital obstruct redistributive policies to curb health inequities (e.g., see Navarro 2007a; Navarro et al. 2006). The vast wealth and power of dominant interest groups promoting neoliberalism sustain health inequities.

Studying health inequities means looking at how different groups within and outside the state and its mechanisms try to shape government policies in their favour. A common mistake is believing that everyone, whether in government or not, has an equal say in making public and health policies. This simplification completely overlooks the uneven power dynamics that influence state policies regarding the social determinants of health inequities.

Some people think that policy actors, like groups in society, businesses, and governments, can work together to agree on health policies. However, they overlook the irreconcilable differences in their interests under capitalism. For example, capitalists habitually oppose workers' demand for decent work and wages. Big real estate companies fiercely fight against socialized housing. Big pharmaceutical companies do not want public drug distribution systems. Also, the plans of the government, shaped by their political party, can go against what other groups and advocates want in terms of laws, economics, cultures, institutions, and health goals. Powerful interest groups, like political and business leaders, control much of the lawmaking processes to benefit themselves, not the public. Less powerful groups dealing with social and health inequities often lose out. We need to replace prevailing social systems that exploit people and the planet.

Note

1   Cathy Crowe, a distinguished member of the Order of Canada, co-founded the Shelter and Housing Justice Network and currently serves as a Distinguished Visiting Practitioner at Toronto Metropolitan University.

CHAPTER FIVE

The Role of Evidence and Ideas

Research equips us with evidence and ideas that can inform political actions and social activism to address health inequities. However, do evidence and research-informed ideas actually influence state policy action? I analyzed insights from my interviewees to determine whether, and if so, to what extent do evidence and ideas influence state policies on health inequities in Canada.

Policy Paradigms and Policy Ideas

Policy paradigms illustrate how ideas affect health policy, suggesting that policymaking is a societal learning process. According to political economist Peter Hall, there are three main points to consider regarding state policymaking: (1) past policies primarily influence current ones; (2) we learn about policies predominantly from experts in specific fields; and (3) governments usually make decisions independently, barely considering what society wants when making policies (1993, 277–78). Thus, policy paradigms and changes in health policy go hand in hand.

An analysis of the policy process underscores three elements: policy goals, instruments used for implementation, and specific settings of these instruments. Policy *goals* set the direction for public policy in areas of interest. The *instruments* of policy are the means used to achieve these goals. The *settings* of these instruments refer to the locations where they are applied (Hall 1993, 278–79). For instance, in addressing health inequities resulting from housing insecurity, the policy goal might be to reduce such insecurity. The instrument could be the provision of social housing, and the setting would be the level at which this housing is made available to achieve the desired health outcomes. These three components of the policy process may result in varying degrees of policy change. Three levels of policy change occur in the following scenarios.

First order change involves making minor policy adjustments without altering the main policy. For example, policymakers revised the minimum lending rate multiple times without fundamentally changing the policy goals. Instead, these were minor tweaks informed by past events and expert future projections (Hall 1993, 278). *Second order change* involves moderate adjustments to achieve the same policy goals. For example, policymakers implemented a new way to control money flow called cash limits for public spending while moving away from rigid monetary growth targets. First and second order changes are different methods to achieve the same policy goals (Hall 1993, 278). Lastly, policy shifted from a Keynesian approach, where the government plays an active role in the economy, to a monetarist perspective. Monetarists believe that economic problems can be fixed without much interference from government. This *third order change* completely transformed various parts of the policy, including tools, patterns, and fundamental principles, making it a radical change (Hall 1993, 279).

Policy paradigms provide a structured way to understand the depth and nature of changes in health policy. For example, the switch from Keynesian to neoliberal policies has brought significant challenges. Chapter 2 explains that this shift resulted in massive cuts to social support, the termination of national housing programs, and the transfer of housing control to lower levels of government. Consequently, housing insecurity and homelessness became widespread. Chapter 3 shows that neoliberalism eroded the public health care system. These policy changes led to a severe health care crisis, with overcrowded hospitals, closures of emergency services, longer wait times, insufficient staffing levels, and negative impacts on workers and patients.

Third order change, also called a *paradigm shift*, is a radical policy change. It is not just about minor or moderate adjustments but instead is a major shift due to societal factors like politics, economics, cultures, and institutions rather than just what experts say. These changes arise from urgent societal problems, leading to the implementation of new policies and, at times, policy failures, which create a whole new way of thinking and doing things. Hall (1993, 290) says:

> Policy paradigms can be seen as one feature of the overall terms of political discourse. They suggest that the policy-making process can be structured by a particular set of ideas, just as it can be structured by a set of institutions. The two often reinforce each other since the routines of policymaking are usually designed to reflect a particular set of ideas about what can and should be done in a sphere of policy.

But the ideas embodied in a policy paradigm have a status somewhat independent of institutions that can be used, as in the case of monetarism, to bolster or induce changes in institutional routines.

Ideas and institutions simultaneously affect health policies, but they can also work separately. Politics is not just about learning but also about who has power. Hall further reminds us that "when policy paradigms become the object of open political contestation, the outcome depends on the ability of each side to mobilize a sufficient electoral coalition in the political arena" (1993, 290) and beyond parliamentary spaces. Changing institutions means changing how people engage in dialogue and action; it involves power struggles among various social forces inside and outside politics or the state's realms.

Power is central to policymaking, and policy advocates influence state policy. While intellectual debates can lead to policy changes, social actions, political movements, and media narratives mainly shape policy discussions. When powerful groups set policy goals, it is difficult for less influential groups to make substantial changes. We need to comprehend both the theory and practice of policymaking because all state policies affect health.

Six Travelling Ideas

Katherine Smith's (2007, 2013a, 2013b, 2014) pioneering studies on how evidence and research-informed ideas influence health policy build on Hall's research on policy paradigms. Smith, a professor of public health policy, analyzes documents and interviews government officials (such as civil servants and ministers) and others (such as academics and researchers) involved in health inequities research and policymaking. Smith identified a trend: although everyone claimed that public policies to address health inequities lacked *evidence*, most agreed that *ideas* still influenced state policy decisions. Ideas travelling toward policy can become successful, partial, fractured, recontextualized, weak, or non-journeys.

- *Successful journeys.* Some ideas exert a strong influence on public policy. For example, policymakers prioritize biomedical approaches (e.g., lifestyle changes) in discussions and actions, even when insufficient evidence supports them. This case demonstrates that "it is ideas, rather than research evidence, which have travelled from research into policy" (Smith 2007, 1438). Health policymaking primarily relies on ideas rather than evidence.

- *Partial journeys.* Some ideas impact public policies, but not entirely. For instance, focusing on economic factors gains attention but does not lead to significant policy changes. The Black Report in the UK pointed out how income affects health, but this idea was "merely at the level of rhetoric" (Smith 2007, 1442). It is difficult to turn specific policy ideas into action.
- *Fractured journeys.* Some ideas break apart as they enter health policy. For example, the psychosocial theory of health inequities, which highlights how stress from living and working conditions or social status affects health, gets fragmented in health policy. Policymakers pay attention to social capital but ignore income inequalities (Smith 2007, 1443; 2013a, 86–87). This selective focus means they miss the point that health inequities come from income gaps, leading to less effective health policies. Thus, it is crucial to fully integrate research into public policy.
- *Re-contextualized journeys.* Early life development was one of the few ideas that made it from research to policy. However, policymakers continue to view lifestyles and behaviours (e.g., smoking and poor diet) and inadequacy of health services as the main reasons for health inequities. This perspective persists even though research on social determinants of health has thoroughly debunked their central role in creating health inequities. These re-interpreted ideas reach policy because policymakers filter research-based ideas to fit "institutionalized ideas (or policy paradigms)" (Smith 2013a, 85–86). This institutional bias affects which policy ideas are accepted, modified, or rejected.
- *Weak journeys.* Some ideas about health inequities hardly affect public policy. Connections between socioeconomic status and health, the impact of culture on behaviour, and the idea that genetics and IQ affect health outcomes have little influence on health discussions and actions (Smith 2013b, 95). Understanding why some ideas about health inequities do not make a significant impact can help us improve policymaking. To make policymaking more transparent and complete, we must reflect on why policymakers prioritize certain policy ideas.
- *Non-journeys.* Some ideas never make it into public policy, such as the political economy of health, which examines how class relations shape economic policies and affect health. Despite their importance, these ideas have not influenced state policies. This lack

of interest stems from the belief among politicians, policymakers, civil servants, academics, advocates, researchers, and funders that these ideas are "'impractical,' 'ideological,' 'radical,' or 'unhelpful'" (Smith 2013b, 98). Because of biases, if not ignorance, valuable ideas are excluded from health policymaking. Determining if ideas get excluded because they are unworkable or due to these biases is crucial.

Institutional barriers like filtering, connectivity, and amnesia shape policy ideas (Smith 2013a, 2013b). Filtering occurs when governmental departments alter ideas, complicating unified health policy. Health departments often ignore non-medical ideas, showing their selectiveness. Weak connections within policy institutions exacerbate filtering. Ministers rely on external advice, and some experts avoid challenging the government. Trust issues and communication gaps between ministers and civil servants prevent the push for sound health policies. Institutional amnesia, due to high turnover, recycles old ideas and perpetuates repetitive research on health inequities, further hindering new policy development (Smith 2013a, 2013b).

Smith (2013a, 2013b) suggests the following for improving health research and policy: (1) policymakers, knowledge brokers, and researchers must collaborate, especially for small policy changes; (2) researchers and academics should engage with politicians, community groups, and the media for broader changes; (3) health research and policymaking should be more closely linked; (4) policy paradigms and institutionalized ideas should be examined to understand how health research and policy connect; and (5) consistent and sufficient funding should be ensured for knowledge brokers. Smith stresses viewing health research and policy as a dynamic "interplay of ideas" and focusing on how ideas, not just evidence, influence policy changes for health equity.

Challenges with the Journeys of Ideas

Many scholars do not provide a straightforward answer to the question: "What are ideas?" Instead, they hint at or assume meanings without defining the term. This lack of clarity in basic concepts can create confusion and hinder effective health research, policy, practice, and advocacy. Therefore, defining "ideas" is crucial for avoiding confusion, particularly in health studies. The six journeys of ideas about health inequity research and policy are problematic to grasp because the terms "ideas," "paradigms," and "ideologies" are ambiguously defined. Hall (1993) and Smith (2007) did not define ideas clearly and sometimes mixed them up with terms like paradigms and ideologies, making it easy to criticize their work constructively. For example, some scholars say, "Ideas and paradigms are ontologically obscure and, therefore, any attempt to draw explanatory leverage and generalizable knowledge will be problematic" (Cairney and Weible 2015, 85). Others state, "Ideas become desiderata, catch-all concepts" (Blyth 1997, 231). Therefore, being transparent about our terminology is imperative. Ensuring precision with our words enables us to translate research into policies and practices. Clearly defining "ideas" will help clarify their meaning.

Some scholars define ideas as "causal beliefs about economic, social, and political phenomena" (Béland and Cox 2016, 230). These scholars see ideas as relational insights, whether they describe something as true or false, tangible or intangible. This definition narrows ideas to a clear cause-and-effect view of phenomena, emphasizing our perceptions of their validity. Others describe ideas as "beliefs, knowledge, worldviews, and shared definitions of policy problems, images, and solutions within groups, organizations, networks, and political systems" (Heikkila and Cairney 2014, 365). Thus, ideas function at individual and communal levels. Ideas are not limited to causal beliefs; they encompass collective worldviews, underpinning how groups perceive and tackle issues, such as health inequities.

The practical use of ideas in policymaking involves contributing to policy discussions, shaping proposals, and creating a common language among policymakers (Cairney and Weible 2015). Ideas play different roles in health policymaking, from generating concepts to communicating them. Although the term "ideas" may seem abstract and its definition varies, ideas are crucial for shaping how people think, converse, and act in society. Understanding the many aspects of ideas is key to seeing how they influence health policy and social change.

Moreover, although ideas and paradigms might seem similar, they have different meanings. In policy, some say a paradigm is a common thought in policy communities. Others define it as "a field of accepted practices that determine the goals, priorities, and content of policy" (Blyth 1997, 237). While ideas can be individual or shared beliefs about phenomena, paradigms are the accepted norms and practices that guide a community or field, such as politics, economics, health policy, or nursing.

Failing to distinguish between ideas and paradigms leads to misconceptions and misunderstandings about the role and influence each holds in health policymaking. However, understanding the difference helps us comprehend their unique impacts on health policy and societal frameworks. While both are influential, they operate in distinct realms, with ideas serving as the building blocks that may, over time, solidify into accepted paradigms. Therefore, ideas are precursors to paradigms.

Ideas, paradigms, and ideologies all have specific meanings. Ideology, for instance, is described as "a more or less coherent set of ideas that lays the groundwork for organized political action, be it to maintain, alter, or challenge the existing power system" (Heywood 2017, 10). Ideology drives social and political actions, often embodying systemic intentions. While these terms may overlap, they each have distinct roles and importance. They cannot merely be substituted or used interchangeably. Although ideas, paradigms, and ideologies are interrelated, they operate on different levels. Ideas are foundational beliefs, paradigms represent accepted norms in a community, and ideologies underpin sociopolitical action. Understanding the differences between these concepts is vital for precise communication, meaningful policy change, and crafting new ways of thinking about and acting on health inequities.

In this book, I define "ideas" as follows: Ideas are rooted in human perception. When we, as human beings, engage with tangible material things through our senses, we generate intangible immaterial forms of thoughts, which we term ideas. The independent variables are the materials, whereas the dependent variables are the ideas. We convey our ideas through various verbal and non-verbal forms of communication. Our ideas encompass perceptions, interpretations, introspections, and expressions derived from the material world. The material conditions of life form the bedrock for a holistic understanding of complex interrelations in society, policy, and health.

The Subordinate Role of Evidence and Research-Informed Ideas

Now that we have grasped what ideas, paradigms, and ideologies mean, let us listen to the insights of my interviewees — academics, advocates, and activists — who are knowledgeable about social and health inequities. I asked the participants in the study two main questions: Why do health inequities persist? Do evidence and research-based ideas matter more in making public policies than the power struggles and politics involved in shaping health policies?

Most of the interviewees agreed that while evidence and research-based ideas influence public policy, they often get overshadowed by power struggles, vested interests, and prevailing ideologies. Most of the interviewees specifically mentioned how ideology, interests, and power play a role.

Power over Evidence and Ideas

The power struggle among groups trying to sway state decisions significantly affects how research and facts shape policies. Although research and information are essential, to achieve fair health outcomes for everyone, we must deal with complex issues involving politics, the economy, cultures, institutions, and society. Diverse policy actors, such as politicians, special interest groups, and the public, have conflicting priorities, affecting how research influences health policy.

A cautionary tale about power and influence in health politics: money leads to power, and power leads to more money. Even though solid research should guide decisions about health equity, the power of money has an enormous impact on state policies compared to the facts. Stewart stated:

> The policy and research should absolutely influence the decisions. But again, the power lies where the money is and the intellect. So even if you do present a strong case through policy research with all the backup of why and pointing out what improvements it would bring to society or the issue, still, money seems to have the influence.

Money plays a significant role in society, making it difficult for politicians or governments to make substantial changes without making businesses unhappy. Such actions might cause a capital strike, where private enterprises stop or reduce their investments. Government officials know that money has much power, and they worry about the adverse reactions they might get if they try to do something that could reduce the power of businesses, like taking over private insurance companies. Professor of sociology William Carroll explained:

> Capital dominates human affairs. And so, even if a politician or political party or government is really wanting to make major changes, it's not easy to do them. It's very difficult

without ruffling the feathers of the business community and possibly precipitating a so-called capital strike. And so, state managers are always aware of the fact that capital holds the trump card, really, in terms of what might happen if a certain policy comes into play, like, say, nationalizing private insurance companies or something like that. Once you make any kind of move in the direction of infringing on the power of capital, there's a big pushback.

Money often has more influence than evidence in health policymaking. However, things can improve when people demand policy decisions based on facts, as seen in struggles against toxic materials like asbestos or in the fight for universal health care. Political activist Sam Gindin, who was research director for the Canadian Auto Workers for twenty-seven years, pointed this out:

> In workplaces, there's a lot of chemical-related diseases. There's a lot of cancer, and it's because, for a corporation, it might be cheaper to use a particular chemical even if it kills workers. So, the only way you can change it is if the workers organize to fight against it. But sometimes they won't because they're worried that if they organize to fight against it, the place may close, and that's happened. So, even the workers themselves might be reluctant to do it. So, suppose you get a good study that shows that this workplace and these chemicals destroyed peoples' health. You can do things with it. We've been able to get rid of asbestos, for example, in car brakes, in using it in homes, and using it anywhere children are near the school walls. That came about because people organized it, and there was enough pressure on the government because everybody cared about their kids. Other people got worried too. Office workers got worried. So, they were able to have some impact, but it still is a small impact. People have to fight over every little thing. So yeah, they're always at a disadvantage. That doesn't change. That's what capitalism is. It's an unequal society ... But if you organize and mobilize, you can win some things. There's no question; we've won things, including the medical system, which the United States doesn't have.

The relationship between evidence, power, and mobilization is complex. Even with sound ideas backed by research, influential people and groups prevent them from becoming state policies. Evidence is not enough; we need groups of people to push for substantial policy change. In a capitalist system, the ruling government blocks or limits policies related to sharing societal resources, like universal health services and community housing.

Interests over Evidence and Ideas

Capital interest groups ignore facts and ideas from research that are not aligned with their interests. For example, neoliberal state policymakers put financial interests first, even though they say they work for what people need. This is evident when the governing authorities enact private housing rules for businesses to earn more profit instead of implementing socialized housing. Writer and retired Ontario Coalition Against Poverty organizer John Clarke explained:

> I don't think governments function in the interests of most people. So yes, it's an expensive proposition in many ways to abandon people on the streets. And in California, it's reaching the point now where they have a public health crisis as a result of the level of destitution that they've created. But the developers don't want social housing. They want to build luxury housing. The speculators and the bankers similarly are not interested in providing truly affordable housing for most people and dealing with the crisis and homelessness. And so, even at incredible social and economic costs, those inequities continue. They should be challenged. They are challenged. And evidence-based research is a vital tool to use in the fight. But the limitations of it have to be understood because we're not up against a system that is fundamentally rational.

There is a struggle between research findings and the interests of the power elite. Although research highlights significant societal and health problems, the rich, powerful, and state managers set the rules. Housing insecurity and homelessness persist because the state prioritizes private property ownership and caters to capitalists, not objective data. Governments only respond to public demands when large groups unite and pressure them, especially if political leaders fear losing power.

Ideology over Evidence and Ideas

Ideology plays a big role in how the state and its agencies decide policies. Even if they seem to be paying attention to research, they often only choose the information that fits their ideological inclinations. Professor Toba Bryant, who specializes in the social determinants of health and health policy, explained how this bias makes it more challenging to create equitable health policies.

> My PhD thesis was all about whether evidence played any role in public housing decisions. I still think this is the case: It's the political ideology, rather, the ideological commitment of government, that really shaped policy. I think they make the decisions; then, they look for the evidence to support their decisions to justify their action or inaction.

Politicians usually stick to their ideology rather than considering evidence in policymaking. Even when scholars, advocates, and activists use facts, the ideas that win often match what the government already thinks. Even if community groups provide evidence, it is hard to change leaders' minds if it contradicts their beliefs. In a capitalist system, decisions based on evidence are rare, especially if those ideas explicitly critique the horrors of capitalism.

Synergy of Power, Interests, and Ideology

Influential groups' power, interests, and ideology prevent what research tells us is needed to address inequities in health and society. This situation arises because the state and its apparatuses ensure big businesses accumulate more capital instead of workers and the public getting good jobs, places to live, and health services.

Trevor Hancock is a retired professor and senior public health and social policy scholar, a former consultant at the Ministry of Health in British Columbia, and the founding leader of the Green Party in Canada and Ontario. Hancock's insight shows that policies hardly change, even with sufficient evidence; politics usually wins, as we see with climate and health issues:

> We have all kinds of evidence, but is it changing policy? Hardly at all. In the US, not at all. In Brazil, not at all. In the Philippines, probably not at all. In Canada, not at all. Why does the NDP government support the LNG [liquid

natural gas] pipelines and LNG industry? Why does the federal government support the Alberta tar sands industry and the pipeline? The evidence that those are bad things to be doing is really quite clear. The evidence that most of the fossil fuel that we have in Canada actually has to stay in the ground if we want to avoid two degrees centigrade warming doesn't really seem to affect policy very much.

Scientists have shown that Big Capital has been causing rapid climate change for a long time, and most agree on what is happening and what will happen because of it. However, despite knowing its dangers, little has been done by capitalist states to address the ecological crisis. This lack of action is due to factors such as profit-making from fossil fuels, political ideology, and public perception, which can slow down or change how quickly and effectively we respond to climate change. Hancock elaborated:

> I often go back to Carol Weiss. Years ago, she said three things that go into the decision making ... information, ideology, and interest. And then she went on to say, don't for one moment think that information can trump either ideology or interest. So if you look at the whole climate debate right now, it's actually an ideological debate. The right-wing, the Republicans, some Conservatives here, their rejection of the evidence has nothing to do with the evidence. It's really an ideology ... our group thinks this way, and we are aligned with the fossil fuel industry because they're rich and powerful. Our whole system is based on cheap energy. And so we have to keep going kind of thing. And bugger the evidence.
>
> And that second one, which is actually very closely related to that, is interest. By interest, she meant power and wealth and stakeholders. So, who gets the policy they want? The people who have the money and power to influence it. So, the fossil fuel industry is very powerful ... And so, no matter what the evidence is, they have a financial interest in not having any controls upon them or having the minimum of controls. And so, that will triumph usually. So, you put together ideology and interest, and it will almost always overcome evidence or information.

Postmodernism's ideas further complicate societal and public health matters. It argues that there is no one truth, which makes it more challenging to make evidence-based decisions. This way of thinking gives power to politicians who make appealing statements with no facts to support them. The concept of relative truth weakens the foundation for making effective policies based on research. The late political scientist Leo Panitch explained:

> It feeds the Trumps and the Dutertes of this world who can use the rejection of truth, the rejection of evidence much more powerfully than those people who say my subjectivity as a Filipino is all that matters: "I know what it is to be oppressed because I'm a Filipino maid." And that's the real truth, but it's not the real truth. I mean, in so far as this is true, it reflects the Filipino maid's experience in the real world, not simply because she's Filipino and a maid. It reflects what she has learned objectively about how the world works. Whereas a lot of people start with: "I'm a Filipino, so I'm oppressed." There are capitalist Filipinos too ... I'm picking on Filipinos. They're the least likely to do it. It's usually the daughters of capitalist Filipinos who come to the university saying: "All I need to know is that I'm an oppressed Filipino." I'm sure you experience this. You hear this much more in Canada, not from Filipinos. You hear it from Indigenous students at universities. You hear it from Black students at universities. You can even hear it from Jewish students at universities who generally don't come from poor families. But all it matters is my subjectivity and my sense of oppression and marginalization or my gendered sense of oppression or my sexual sense of oppression. This detracts from the validity of evidence-based research. Imagine if Marx hadn't spent all that time in the British Museum studying the evidence-based nature of capitalism, and all he did was say capitalism is bad.

We must listen to people's stories and understand their challenges, but relying on personal experiences without considering scientific data can lead to ignoring essential facts needed for effective policy ideas. Powerful groups might use these personal stories to ignore what is true for everyone and push their self-serving agendas. Therefore, balancing personal experiences and objective facts is vital when discussing society's problems and crafting health policies.

The power of evidence and ideas for new policies depends heavily on what the state and big businesses want. Consequently, scholars, advocates, activists, and people working to change policies have a tough job influencing state decisions to achieve health for all. Greg Albo talked about how challenging this fight is.

> I think the role of an honest researcher, an honest scholar, a socially committed scholar, and one who's in at the end of the day for following wherever the evidence-based policy leads one is to conclude that if there are obstacles in the way, how do we remove those obstacles to follow up with [what] the policies tell us to do? And then that ranges us into a participatory research agenda and participatory forms of politics because it's only by combining that evidence with participatory forms of politics, collective forms of mobilization, that we can take the policies' outcomes in the direction that the evidence is pointing us to. And therefore, it's understanding evidence-based policy not in the narrow sense or science-based policy in the narrow sense but by pulling it up that the science is telling us this is a structural policy and structural policy limit. And therefore, the evidence points us to finding ways to remove that obstacle. And that's when politics and participation start becoming important. And that's where the hardcore of the state and the hardcore of inequality start limiting those choices.

Science tells us we need significant societal and health policy changes to improve lives. However, the current state of politics, cultures, institutions, and the economy prevents us from discussing and acting to change the status quo. To overcome these formidable challenges and achieve fair health for everyone, people must get involved in research and activism in their workplaces, communities, and governments. The following five crucial points need to be borne in mind in the fight for health equity: First, evidence only matters if it aligns with what Big Capital and political elites want or if they can twist it to fit their needs. Second, the state and its apparatuses care more about making money and keeping the capitalist system thriving than using evidence. They only use evidence if it supports the capitalist way of life running smoothly. Third, ruling governments might sometimes use policy ideas supported by research that counter their interests and ideologies, but only, as we have emphasized earlier, if they feel pressured by the public, unmasking them as flawed and illegitimate. Fourth, capital power, interests, and ideology have a more significant impact on health policies than we previously thought, suggesting that decisions are not mainly based on research and evidence. Lastly, despite the belief that institutionalized ideas or policy paradigms shape health policies, the mix of power, interests, and ideology drives them.

CHAPTER SIX

A Critical Political Economy Approach

Inspired by Engels (1845), Marx and Engels ([1848] 1964), and Marx (1867) and building on my own works (Borras 2021, 2022, 2023), this study examines avoidable health inequities through a critical political economy lens. The critical political economy approach to health inequities views social and health inequities as tangible, interconnected, and subject to change. It posits that human beings are inherently social, with lives shaped by the social relations of production. These relations underpin social structures such as the economy, politics, and law, influencing social consciousness, which emerges from material and social conditions of life. Social conflict arises when social forces clash within existing social relations, resolving through societal revolution that transforms social structures and creates a new societal order.

The critical political economy approach to health inequities accounts for economic, political, cultural, institutional, environmental, and historical forces and factors affecting human and planetary health. It scrutinizes how capitalism, infused with colonialism, racism, and sexism, shapes unequal health outcomes. It focuses on how ideology, interests, and power determine who gets healthy and who does not. The critical political economy approach examines how integrally imbricated social relations like class, race, and gender affect resource production, distribution, and consumption. It investigates conflicts between governments, businesses, and civil society organizations, including workers' and people's movements, in shaping health policies. It reveals power dynamics and their influence on the allocation of the social determinants of health, resulting in health inequities. The critical political economy approach examines how human-to-human and human-to-nature relations impact health outcomes, emphasizing wealth and power distribution to understand health disparities. It not only identifies problems but also suggests solutions, offering scholars, advocates, activists, practitioners, and policymakers tools to address the root causes of health inequities. The goal is to create a better society where everyone can live a healthy life and reach their full potential.

Capitalism and Its Impact on Health

Capitalism is a political-economic system that views virtually everything — even essential human needs — as a potential commodity. In this setup, everyone — from workers selling their labour to capitalists seeking profits — is tied to the market's dynamics. At the heart of capitalism is the drive for profit and continual wealth accumulation (Wood 2017, 2–3). Such a perspective pushes capitalists toward an endless loop: maximizing profit, gathering wealth, and reinvesting capital for further financial gains. This ongoing cycle comes at a tremendous cost, especially when examining its impact on ecology, society, and people's lives.

During our interview, Sam Gindin discussed how workers face severe challenges in societies that follow the capitalist system. They often get paid less and have to function like machines, adversely affecting their well-being. Because workers do not come together as a class, it is tough for them to stand up against this exploitative system. Gindin suggests that if workers unite and act together, they can better address socioeconomic and health inequities rooted in capitalism.

> Capitalism. That's the story ... This is what it means to live in a class society. It's unequal for workers, which means not just lower wages, but the pace of work is constantly tightened, which puts pressure on people. It means they live in permanent insecurity, which has all kinds of health and mental health issues ... It's the basic workings of our capitalist society of one-half of the equation. The second half of the equation is that we haven't been able to build the kind of social forces that have effectively offset that. I think an obvious answer, it's about class and the relative balance of class forces. And the fact that workers aren't a class, they're fragmented individuals, and as fragmented individuals, they don't have the power to take on the capitalist system, inequalities. And the working class over the last 30, 40 years now has been defeated. So, it's no surprise that we find these results.

Panitch's insights further confirm why some people have more societal advantages, including better health. The main reason behind these inequities is the capitalist system, where the state and its rules ensure class relations and a power balance tilted in favour of capitalists getting richer and richer at the expense of the workers. Government policy can make these inequities better or worse. Although public policies may sometimes produce meaningful outcomes, the real problem is that in capitalism, wealth accumulation precedes people's health.

> In one word, the answer to your question is capitalism, which is not a product of government policy but rather is the nature of the social system, a socioeconomic system in which government policy is located. So, the fundamental parameters of inequalities in a country like Canada are given by capitalist social relations and the requirements of reproducing favourable conditions for capital accumulation and reproducing the class relations that are necessary for a capitalist society. That's my fundamental answer. That said, it's obvious, the case that government policy, which is a reflection of the balance of social forces in a society given periods of time and particular conjuncture, the government policy can modify, ameliorate, exacerbate this fundamental inequality, which are systemic.

Gindin's and Panitch's views are not new. In capitalist societies, the working class and those living in poverty have consistently encountered more health challenges than the affluent and capitalist class. The grim conditions of nineteenth-century factories, where workers endured extended hours in unsafe environments for meagre wages (Engels 1845), stand as testimony. This trend persisted in the twentieth century, when workers bore higher risks for exhaustion, mental stress, and exposure to toxic substances, resulting in increased injuries and fatalities (Navarro 1986, 106–40). Even in the twenty-first century, workers suffer from black lung disease, which reduces life expectancy by over twelve years (Mazurek et al. 2018, 820). Historical patterns show that class relations in capitalism have always been the prime mover of health inequities.

In capitalist societies, many working-class families and people experiencing poverty cannot afford necessities such as nutritious food, quality housing, and health services due to insufficient earnings. This class inequality leads to the rich and capitalists typically living longer than their counterparts. Capitalism inherently prioritizes profit maximization and capital accumulation, often at the expense of lives. Big Capital kills on a massive scale.

Neoliberalism, Work, and Health

Neoliberal policies have had severe effects on the workforce, leading to a massive rise in informal workers worldwide, totalling more than 2 billion. One adverse result of this neoliberal trend is the proliferation of the *precariat* — workers who have unstable jobs and often live in poverty. These precarious workers typically hold temporary or part-time jobs (Standing 2014, 10). Manual labourers, young people, those with limited education, immigrants, and women are most affected. Besides financial problems, these workers also face serious health risks (Benach et al. 2016; Muntaner et al. 2010).[1] Instead of improving conditions for workers, neoliberal capitalism has exacerbated challenges both at work and in life.

Socioeconomic and health inequities are inherent outcomes of capitalism. These inequities arise because the bourgeoisie, who own the means of production, focus on maximizing profits, resulting in the concentration of national wealth in the hands of monopoly capitalists. As capital accumulates wealth for the few, it simultaneously generates intense labour exploitation, brutality, ignorance, misery, and mental degradation for the many (Marx, 1867, 451). Addressing health inequities within capitalist societies becomes exceedingly challenging due to these deeply entrenched economic structures and priorities.

Capital accumulation is inversely related to economic and health equity. Unequal class relations can be seen concretely in wealth and health inequities. For instance, the *Executive Excess 2023* report reveals an outrageous earnings gap in a hundred large companies, collectively known as the Low-Wage 100. CEOs in these firms earned an average of 603 times more than a typical worker, taking home $15.3 million compared to the worker's $31,672 annually in 2022 (Anderson 2023, 1–3). This income inequality arises at the expense of the health of workers.

Consider Amazon, one of the world's largest corporations, with a roughly $1.5 trillion market value and 1.5 million workers. Amazon warehouse workers experience higher risks of back injuries and other musculoskeletal problems. These risks result from lifting heavy items, prolonged hours of demanding tasks, and sending workers with potential back injuries or concussions back to work without proper medical assessments (US Department of Labor 2023a, 2023b). Capitalist labour practices exacerbate injuries, resulting in long-term suffering. In 2020, the rate of injuries at Amazon was 6.5 per 100 workers, compared to 4 per 100 in non-Amazon warehouses. Its serious injury rate was 80% higher than other companies (Strategic Organizing Center 2023, 3–5). Workplace injury is not coincidental but indicative of a systemic issue in capitalism, where prioritizing profit over worker safety is inherent. In a capitalist system, the driving force is capital accumulation, not the well-being of people.

Neoliberalism enabled the wealthiest 1% to amass even more cultural, political, and economic power (Carroll and Sapinski 2018). For instance, while most working families in Canada saw little income growth, the ultra-rich, the top 0.01%, experienced a 145% increase in their incomes from 1990 to 2010 (Peters 2012, 19). This inequality arose as union membership declined, weakening workers' bargaining power and resulting in diminishing real wages and reduced benefits. Moreover, the proliferation of temporary and part-time jobs supplanted full-time employment. Large companies laid off workers to boost profits, resulting in widespread unemployment, poverty, and housing insecurity as corporate downsizing and small business closures became common (Banting and Myles 2013; Finkel 2018; McBride and Shields 1996; Peters 2012). Big Capital exerted dominance over workers' movements and increasingly influenced state policymakers to enact policies favouring themselves and their associates.

In 2016, Canada's top 87 affluent families — mostly big capitalists — had as much wealth as the 12 million poorest people in Canada. Their wealth was nearly equivalent to the combined wealth of individuals in Prince Edward Island, Newfoundland and Labrador, and New Brunswick. This extreme wealth inequality stems from several factors: higher earners save and invest more, wealthy families benefit from having top-paid CEOs, and generational wealth transfer plays a crucial role. Additionally, the tax system favours capital gains and dividends over wages and allows tax avoidance through private corporations and tax havens (Macdonald 2018, 5–10).

In 2019, the wealth distribution in Canada and the United States exhibited notable similarities. In the US, the top 1% of the population held 35.7% of the nation's wealth. In comparison, the top 1% in Canada controlled 26% of the country's wealth, although Statistics Canada reported a lower estimate of 17.3%. Additionally, the wealthiest 0.1% of Americans owned 16.2% of the total wealth, whereas the Canadian counterparts held 12.4%, with official figures suggesting it was just 3.9% (Skilleter 2024, 1).

Wealth inequality in Canada has been increasing, with the top 20% of households owning more than two-thirds (67.6%) of the country's net worth as of early 2024, averaging $3.4 million per household. In contrast, the bottom 40% of households collectively held only 2.8% of the wealth, averaging $70,356 each. The disparity between the wealth of the bottom 40% and the top 20% widened by 0.3 percentage points from the previous year, reaching 64.8%. This growing gap is primarily due to the wealthiest individuals benefitting from a 5.3% rise in financial asset values, which offset a 0.7% drop in real estate values. The wealthiest households had 58.4% of their assets in financial investments, while the least wealthy had only 28.8% in such assets during this period (Statistics Canada 2024b, 4). Unsurprisingly, men and women with the lowest incomes live about 8.1 and 3.6 years less, respectively, than those with the highest incomes (Milligan and Schirle 2018, 19). Neoliberal capitalism creates and perpetuates class inequality and, in turn, health inequities.

Capitalism–Imperialism–Colonialism–Racism Nexus

Colonialism began in the 1500s when European nations took over other lands and people primarily through military force. After World War II, many countries fought for national liberation and independence, leading to less direct control by European powers. However, Indigenous groups, especially in places with European settlers, still face challenges in protecting their traditional lands. Ongoing settler colonialism in Canada and other parts of the world involves horrific crimes against humanity, such as genocide, with its effects still being felt today.

Colonialism has evolved into neocolonialism, where powerful nations exert indirect control rather than direct territorial conquest. This form of dominance severely impacts the economies, politics, cultures, and institutions of the Global South while benefiting the Global North. Neocolonialism operates in tandem with capitalism, as large corporations and powerful states, led by the imperialist United States, use their wealth and influence through global finance, economic policies, and military threats to dominate other countries.

Throughout history, the intertwining practices of colonialism, capitalism, and imperialism have profoundly impacted global economies and human well-being. Modern capitalism originated between 1500 and 1800, influenced by imperial and colonial practices that extended state power internationally. This period saw the accumulation of merchant capital from natural resources and agricultural products like sugar and cotton, often through the labour of enslaved peoples (Veltmeyer 2020, 3–8). In the nineteenth century, the close relationship between international markets and the capitalist mode of production became evident — the need for capital accumulation intensified labour exploitation, especially of enslaved peoples. This phenomenon is exemplified by the colonization of America, where the subjugation of Indigenous and Black populations fueled the ascent of capitalist production on both domestic and global scales.[2] This expansion, driven by the pursuit of resources like gold and silver (Marx 1867, 164, 533), propelled industries forward while communities and people suffered.

Nancy Fraser (2023, xv) says that "'capitalism' refers not to a type of economy but to a type of *society*." She calls it "an institutionalized societal order" (19) and delineates the four stages of capitalism: mercantile capitalism, liberal-colonial capitalism, state-managed capitalism, and financialized capitalism. Understanding these stages helps to contextualize the evolving nature of capitalist society.

Mercantile capitalism — sixteenth to eighteenth century — was driven primarily by expropriation rather than exploitation.[3] During this period, land enclosures in Europe and the conquest and enslavement in Africa and the Americas were common, overshadowing later factory worker exploitation and shaping social hierarchies. Early racial distinctions like "Europeans" versus "natives" and "whites" versus "blacks" were less pronounced since most non-property owners lacked political rights. Dependency was the norm without its later associated stigma. The sharp contrast between "free" and "subject" races became evident when political struggles granted liberal rights to male European workers. This shift, along with factory exploitation, led to the firm establishment of the white supremacist order of modern capitalism, marking the transition to liberal-colonial capitalism (41–42). Mercantile capitalism laid the groundwork for contemporary racial and economic inequalities and health inequities.

In the nineteenth century, mercantile capitalism evolved into liberal-colonial capitalism, interconnecting expropriation and exploitation. European colonial rule, the US dispossession of Indigenous Peoples and racialized slavery persisted during this era. This phase, characterized by large-scale manufacturing and class conflicts, fueled democratic struggles. These struggles resulted in citizenship rights for European workers while suppressing anti-colonial efforts. Consequently, racial distinctions sharpened, creating the free "white" worker and the dependent racialized subject, embedding modern racism in capitalism. In this era, expropriation and exploitation, though seemingly separate, were systematically imbricated, with colonial expropriation fueling industrial exploitation in the capitalist core. Both processes drove global capital accumulation (42–43). Liberal-colonial capitalism entrenched racial and economic inequalities by intertwining colonial expropriation with industrial exploitation, shaping health inequities.

In the era of state-managed capitalism, expropriation and exploitation became deeply entangled. Racialized workers in the capitalist core, paid less than whites, experienced both. Notably, African Americans, displaced by mechanization, joined the workforce as second-class workers under Jim Crow laws, with poor wages and denied citizenship. Welfare states protected workers but marginalized minorities, sparking civil rights protests in the 1960s. Independence struggles in the decolonizing periphery aimed to elevate ex-colonial subjects, but many remained vulnerable due to unequal global trade. Post-colonial states also expropriated Indigenous populations. Distinct forms persisted: people of colour often faced expropriation, while whites were typically exploited, but hybrid cases of simultaneous expropriation and exploitation emerged (43–45). State-managed capitalism perpetuated racial-economic and health inequities by tightly interweaving expropriation and exploitation, disproportionately affecting subjugated groups.

In today's era of financialized global capitalism, expropriation and exploitation closely intertwine and spread extensively. Industrial exploitation shifts to BRICS countries — Brazil, Russia, India, China, and South Africa — while expropriation surpasses exploitation in profit generation. Debt pressures states to collude with investors, resulting in widespread dispossession. Peasants and post-colonial populations face intensified corporate land grabs and sovereign debt, exacerbating their expropriation. In the historic core, precarious service work replaces unionized labour, reducing wages and merging expropriation with exploitation. Welfare-state cuts further marginalize workers. Offloading services onto families primarily impacts women in precarious work. Austerity measures erode labour rights and increase consumer debt, targeting racialized borrowers with hyper-expropriative loans (45–48). Financialized capitalism exacerbates social and health inequities by deeply imbricating expropriation and exploitation on a global scale, heightening the vulnerabilities of marginalized populations.

Financialized capitalism blurs the line between free workers and defenceless subjects, with the "expropriated and exploited citizen-worker" becoming the norm. Despite this, the continuum remains racialized, disproportionately affecting people of colour. In the US, Black and brown Americans experience high rates of subprime loan foreclosures and plant closures, leading to deteriorating public services. Black men are heavily impacted by harsh imprisonment and coerced labour (47–48). Financialized capitalism perpetuates racialized health inequities, particularly through the economic and social marginalization of people of colour.

Health inequities exist and persist in all phases of capitalism. Under capitalism, whatever its particular manifestation, exploited and expropriated people and communities continue to suffer. The enduring impacts of imperialism and colonialism on the mental health and well-being of colonized peoples are well-documented. The emotional pain and physical harm inflicted by imperialist colonizers have led to numerous mental health problems and early deaths (Fanon 1963). The cruelty of capitalism, combined with oppressive systems like slavery, serfdom, and racialization, has caused severe health inequities.

Capitalism–Colonialism Nexus and Health Divide

Bryan Palmer (2023) stated: "Capitalism and colonialism are the undeniable foundations of modern Canada." Settler colonialism and capitalism led to the forced assimilation and disruption of Indigenous ways of life. For instance, the mandate of the residential schools was to destroy Indigenous children's cultural identities, and the Indian Act of 1876 confiscated lands and disrupted Indigenous economic and social life. The colonial government also relocated the Inuit into permanent settlements, causing severe health issues (OHRC 2005; Smylie and Firestone 2016). Efforts to rectify these injustices persist amid ongoing trauma in Indigenous communities and people's lives.

In the twenty-first century, Indigenous Peoples continue to face serious social and health problems. They often live in poverty, struggle to access health care, and experience high rates of mental health issues (Anderson et al. 2006; Bailey et al. 2017; Nelson and Wilson 2017). Additionally, Indigenous communities have greater difficulty obtaining sufficient food, securing stable housing, and dealing with homelessness compared to non-Indigenous people. These long-standing issues underscore the marginalization of Indigenous communities.

The interplay of capitalism, imperialism, and colonialism has led to shorter life expectancies for Indigenous Peoples, with disparities of over ten years between the residents of Nunavut and British Columbia (Statistics Canada 2018, 1). Addressing such inequities, requires more than just recognizing these differences in health; we need to fight for a society based on social justice. This means challenging and resisting capitalism, imperialism, and colonialism — social systems that are distinct but integrally intertwined.

Capitalism–Racism Nexus and Health Divide

Racism is deeply entwined with social, economic, and political dynamics (Gilroy 2021), leading to cultural misrecognition, political misrepresentation, economic maldistribution, and health inequities (Borras 2021). Racialized health inequities stem from structural racism rooted in colonial ideas and practices such as settler colonialism and white supremacy. However, structural racism extends beyond beliefs, influencing politics, institutions, and the economy, leading to health disparities among various groups (NCCDH 2018). Neocolonialism, racism, and capitalism constitutively create health inequities. They are not just linked; under capitalism in all its manifestations, neocolonialism and racism are part and parcel of the same system, often expressed in differing manifestations.

Evidence demonstrates that non-racialized communities generally possess more wealth and enjoy better health than other ethnic groups. Even before the pandemic, Indigenous, Black, and Hispanic people faced higher rates of unemployment, poverty, and health issues such as diabetes and heart disease. Asians reported higher stress levels (Bailey et al. 2017). These racialized health inequities are rooted in the capitalist system that consistently undervalues these groups (Borras 2021), many of whom have connections to former colonies worldwide.

The COVID-19 pandemic has further exposed how the co-constitutive character of colonialism, racism, and capitalism contribute to health inequities. Age-adjusted data shows that white individuals had lower COVID-19 death rates compared to Black, Pakistani, and Bangladeshi individuals, even after accounting for disability and sociodemographics (Office for National Statistics n.d.). These disparities are rooted in long-standing inequalities in wealth and economic opportunities, leading to unequal health outcomes. There is a strong link between COVID-19 and financial situations of racialized groups: many who contract the virus live in low-income areas with unstable housing and limited resources, which are often populated by racialized immigrants (Chung et al. 2020). The effects of colonial history on health disparities are evident, as Indigenous and racialized minority groups experience higher rates of infections, hospitalizations, and deaths.

Migrant workers face numerous challenges and unfair treatment, such as not getting paid correctly and being robbed by paying into the employment insurance fund without being able to collect from it. During COVID-19 lockdowns, many struggled to access food, money, and essential information. They are often pressured to work long hours under threats, racism, and constant surveillance. Sadly, many labour laws do not protect migrant workers, leaving them without fair pay or the right to bargain collectively. Moreover, their temporary status and lack of citizenship deter them from standing up for their rights (Migrant Workers Alliance for Change 2020). Without permanent residency or citizenship, most migrants are afraid to demand better working conditions, housing, or health services.

At the Cargill meat plant, almost a thousand migrant workers contracted COVID-19. Despite the severity of the situation, the government and the company reopened the plant after just two weeks. Most workers at this plant are temporary foreign workers from China, Vietnam, and primarily the Philippines (Dryden and Rieger 2020). These workers, coming from areas with colonial histories, were disproportionately affected by the crisis. The Cargill incident exposes neocolonial practices and systemic racism embedded within capitalism, significantly influencing the disproportionate impacts of COVID-19 on different populations. In many industries, the capitalist state and big businesses collude to prioritize profit, often to the detriment of subjugated minorities. This disparity is particularly evident in the treatment of racialized migrant workers within capitalist food systems, wherein their well-being is routinely sacrificed.

Colonized and racialized communities face health inequities for several reasons: (1) forced displacement from ancestral lands; (2) extra challenges in finding jobs, housing, and education; (3) limited access to culturally respectful health services; (4) systemic and individual racism; (5) chronic stress harming their bodies; (6) trauma from colonialism and racism; and (7) exposure to harmful environments (NCCDH 2018).

Low-income and racially marginalized neighbourhoods face more environmental hazards due to segregation, biased zoning, and corporate interests. Practices like biased eminent domain and flawed urban renewal worsen health risks for these communities (Taylor 2014). Environmental racism, driven by capitalism, has created toxic areas like Silicon Valley and Chemical Valley, perpetuating health inequities for racialized groups. Contrary to the biomedical model aligned with capital ideology, individual behaviour and genetics are not the primary drivers of these inequities.

Racialized health inequities result from unequal relations within economic, political, cultural, and institutional systems. Racism is not an isolated phenomenon but an integral part of capitalism, intertwined with colonialism. The capitalist class's pursuit of cheap materials and labour globally, coupled with inadequate capitalist state responses to race, ethnicity, and Indigeneity-related inequalities, intensifies health inequities. Addressing racialized health inequities requires more than just tackling racism alone; it necessitates challenging the co-constitutive systems of racism, neocolonialism, imperialism, and capitalism.

Capitalism–Sexism Nexus and Health Divide

Heteropatriarchy is fundamentally entangled with capitalism, exploiting sex and gender identities for profit and capital accumulation. Reflecting on the nineteenth century underscores the adverse effects of the capitalist mode of production: "Women made unfit for child-bearing, children deformed, men enfeebled, limbs crushed, whole generations wrecked, afflicted with disease and infirmity, purely to fill the purses of the bourgeoisie" (Engels 1845, 123). As technology advanced, machines replace manual labour, prompting capitalists to prefer cheaper female and child labour. Some men even became slave traders, selling their family members to capitalists. Consequently, working-class families were commodified (Marx 1867, 272). Today, capitalism, combined with sexist practices, continues to significantly influence family structures.

The combination of capitalism and sexism rooted in traditional gender roles perpetuates economic disparities between men and women. Studies show a 28% global pay gap between men and women across 104 countries (Boniol et al. 2019, 1). Despite efforts to address these inequalities, progress remains slow, with global pay equity projected to take 136 years to achieve (Oxfam 2022, 4). The capitalist class and capitalist state benefit from cheapening female labour.

Gender discrimination in Canada remains prevalent, with women earning 8.5% less than men in 2023, even after adjusting for various factors.[4] Recent immigrants also face wage discrimination, earning 8% less than Canadian-born workers. Though average wages in the public and private sectors appear similar, significant discriminatory pay gaps exist. In the private sector, men earn 10% more than women, whereas the gender pay gap in the public sector is 5%. Women in the public sector earn 4% more than their private sector counterparts, while men's wages are slightly lower, narrowing the gap (Macdonald 2024, 4–6). Gender and immigrant wage inequalities persist, with public sector practices slightly reducing the gap.

Furthermore, women face a "motherhood penalty," while men benefit from a "fatherhood premium" of 15% in the private sector and 7% in the public sector. The public sector's impact on gender pay equity is most significant among middle- to middle-low income earners, who achieved pay equity at around $20 per hour in 2023. However, at higher income levels, the gender pay gap widens in both sectors, and public sector workers earn less than their private sector peers (Macdonald 2024, 4–6). The public sector also reduces the pay gap for new Canadians, who earn 8% less in the private sector but only 3% less in the public sector than Canadian-born workers (Macdonald 2024, 4–6). Parenthood, income, and migration status affect wage differentials, with the public sector showing better pay equity for middle-income earners and new Canadians than the private sector.

While average hourly pay is similar in both sectors, the public sector addresses discriminatory pay gaps more effectively by raising wages for mothers, women, and new Canadians and lowering wages for fathers, men, medical professionals, and executives. Conversely, the private sector exacerbates discrimination and increases high-end wages (Macdonald 2024, 4–6). The public sector effectively reduces pay gaps for marginalized groups, suggesting its practices could reduce income inequality and poverty.

The entrenched sexism in capitalist workplaces results in heightened challenges for women, including financial, physical, mental, and psychosocial difficulties. Long before the COVID-19 pandemic, the shift from Keynesian to neoliberal policies and the dismantling of the welfare state exacerbated gender and class inequalities. Neoliberalism weakened support systems, especially for women already facing significant challenges. As a result, women and girls have experienced increased gender-based violence (Morrow et al. 2004). Economic policies impact health differently based on gender.

The COVID-19 further exposed the influence of heteropatriarchy on economic and health inequities. Women experienced more significant income losses than men, partly because more women work in health and social work industries with substantial pay gaps and low wages, sectors severely affected by the pandemic. School and care service closures increased unpaid care work, primarily shouldered by women (International Labour Organization 2020). Additionally, domestic violence spiked due to job losses, disrupted support systems, and lockdowns trapping women with abusers, exacerbated by reduced access to reproductive health and legal services (WHO 2020). The pandemic worsened existing gender inequalities, particularly in employment, unpaid care work, and domestic violence.

Similar to how race and ethnicity impact health, gender and class also significantly shape health inequities. These factors are deeply woven into societal systems and affect overall health. Capitalism, which favours certain societal norms, further exploits women, girls, and non-heterosexual men for profit maximization and capital accumulation. Their issues often get ignored, both at work and elsewhere. To hasten progress in health justice, we must fight capitalism, not just sexism. Capitalism co-constitutes heteropatriarchal sexism and remains a primary driver of gendered health inequities.

The Intricate Web of Capitalism-Colonialism-Racism-Sexism

Capitalism, co-constituting colonialism, racism, and sexism, creates a complex societal system that results in and sustains health inequities. In capitalism, factors like race, ethnicity, Indigeneity, sex, and gender are used on purpose to guarantee maximum profits for the capitalists. This deliberate action is evident when examining how the job market functions.

For example, in 2019, the unemployment rate for racialized groups in Canada was 9.2%, compared to 7.3% for non-racialized groups (Block, Galabuzi, and Tranjan 2019, 4). These statistics indicate unequal employment opportunities and suggest a preference among capitalists for hiring non-racialized individuals. Consequently, some business owners exploit the desperation of racialized individuals by offering low wages. In an underground economy, employers bypass legal employment standards by paying workers under the table. Vulnerable workers often accept these arrangements to avoid taxes and increase their immediate income and cash flow to survive.

It is also no accident that Filipino workers earned only 74 cents for every dollar earned by non-Indigenous, non-racialized workers, reflecting a substantial 26% pay gap in 2021 (Statistics Canada 2022c, 2). When considering both race and gender, the gap is even more pronounced: racialized women earned just 59 cents for every dollar earned by non-racialized men (Block, Galabuzi, and Tranjan 2019, 5). These pay differences reveal deeper systemic issues, in which exploitation and expropriation create unequal work opportunities, leading to health inequities. Research has shown that a stable job with good pay leads to a healthier life, and the reverse is also true.

Even in health care, where caring for sick people should be the primary goal, unfair biases still exist. In Western countries, such as the UK, the US and Canada, the capitalist organization of the health care system reflects broader societal divisions. Most doctors, who are at the top, are white men from wealthier families. Nurses, who do much hands-on care, often come from middle to lower-income families. Support staff usually come from working-class backgrounds. This hierarchy perpetuates unfair treatment and affects workers' well-being (Navarro 1977, 446). In Canada, where most of the health care industry is public and not-for-profit, these asymmetrical power relations within health care settings hinder care workers' personal, professional, and financial growth.

As an immigrant from a racialized background who has worked in the health care industry, I witnessed harsh realities. Many health care workers from former colonies are deskilled and their education is unrecognized, resulting in their working primarily in low-paying positions. Deskilling and credential non-recognition are not due to low-quality education or work experience from their origin countries but rather stem from a colonial and capitalist way of thinking and acting that perpetuates exploitation and expropriation. In long-term care, where many workers are racialized women, low pay forces many to work multiple jobs to get by. Long-term care facilities also face constant staff shortages, heavy workloads, abuse, and even violence, all of which harm health. Even worse, those in power normalize these toxic working conditions.

Unfortunately, the government, business, academia, and media usually focus on abuses by care workers while ignoring or hiding the systemic abuses that workers face from residents, families, managers, administrators, and owners. This bias shows an imbalance in the conversation and action, with health care workers' well-being and safety not getting enough attention. The problems in the health care sector sustain inequities based on class, race, and gender.

The COVID-19 pandemic further exposed how unfair the health care system can be, worsening health inequities. Racialized health care workers faced a higher risk; for example, most of the first doctors and health care workers who died from the virus were from racialized communities (Nagpaul 2020). This reality shows a clear connection between health inequities and workers' jobs: racialized workers mainly work directly with patients, while non-racialized workers have administrative roles (GOV.UK 2023). This employment arrangement in capitalist societies reflects wider inequities based on race and ethnicity.

The COVID-19 pandemic also revealed the weaknesses in Canada's long-term care system. Sharleen Stewart highlighted how race, ethnicity, gender, and class all play a part in making life harder for people, especially in migration, education, housing, and health care. She did not directly talk about sexism, racism, neocolonialism, or capitalism, but her observations illustrate how difficult it can be for groups that are experiencing exploitation and expropriation:

> It all points to and lands on communities of colour without a doubt. And that's where you see many immigrants landing in communities of colour. And the majority of those communities are in areas that struggle with, exactly what you say, housing issues ... Child and adult education is, you see, at a lower standard in those communities. The primary example is what's happening right now during this pandemic. I'm calling for a study to be done on exactly that. Let's start doing some demographics on the number of people who got infected and who have died. Do they come from an identified community like ethnicity, race, or gender? I think you're finding that even with our personal support workers who died, they were all women, women of colour ... The workers that we represent, especially in long-term care, the majority of them are women of colour, and they are the lowest paid in the public system. They have a large amount of precarious work where they cannot secure a full-time job. Some of them have worked for a couple of decades in their positions, and they still don't have full-time employment. So, very low-paid, very little benefits, very little retirement security.

The combination of capitalism, neocolonialism, racism, and sexism creates a system where some people have more opportunities and better health than others. These systemically imbricated societal systems unequally affect the working classes, people with low incomes, certain races and ethnicities, Indigenous communities, women, and other genders. Consequently, it is more difficult for these classes and groups to access good health services, healthy food, stable housing, and secure jobs. The COVID-19 pandemic made life even worse for these groups.

Many studies have examined inequities in health and health care, but these significant problems persist despite state interventions.[5] This chapter demonstrates a new approach to understanding the political economy of health inequities based on how class, gender, and race relations affect health. It shows that the unequal distribution of wealth and power is the main reason for these inequities, especially between different classes. It also explains how race and gender play a role in maintaining these differences. To achieve health for all, we must dismantle the capitalist system entangled with neocolonialism, racism, and sexism.

Tackling health inequities requires workers, scholars, activists, and the masses to get involved. We must advocate strongly for policies that distribute wealth evenly, close the gap in pay between genders of different races, and confront how big corporations and state actors work together to protect private over public interests. Overcoming this capital state alliance means workers and communities coming together to share information, teach others, speak up, organize, and mobilize the public. It is about forcing societal changes to free the exploited and oppressed peoples. Such collective action relentlessly fights against capitalism and moves towards a new system and a way of life where everyone gets treated more equally to foster human, societal, and ecological development. This alternative path to health equity is socialism. But what is socialism in the twenty-first century?

Notes

1   Even before the concept of the *precariat*, precarious work was crucial for capitalist domination and capital accumulation. Historically, workers engaged in unstable seasonal agricultural and daily urban jobs. Today, gig economy platforms like Crowdsource, Care.com, and Uber perpetuate job insecurity, lack of benefits, and unstable incomes (De Stefano 2016). The rise of temporary and contract work across industries such as IT and health care allows companies to cut costs and increase flexibility, leading to precarity and its adverse health outcomes.

2   Slavery involved white women, who profited significantly, handling nearly a third of transactions and 40% of trading enslaved women. Enslaved women were valuable for intergenerational wealth, making slavery economically beneficial for both white men and women (Logan 2024). Socioeconomic and health inequities extend beyond gender and race, with class relations being a core aspect.

3   Expropriation, the forcible seizure of wealth from marginalized and subjugated groups, is a fundamental aspect of capitalism, contrary to the belief that it contradicts exploitation. Both expropriation and exploitation fuel capital accumulation, albeit through different mechanisms. Exploitation transfers value to capital via seemingly equitable contractual agreements, where workers receive wages for their labour, covering their living expenses, while capitalists claim surplus labour time. Expropriation involves outright confiscating assets, such as labour, land, minerals, and energy, often with little or no compensation. This practice reduces production costs and boosts profits. Far from being separate, expropriation and exploitation are interdependent. Wage labourers process stolen raw materials with machinery powered by expropriated energy. Their wages are kept low due to the availability of food grown on seized lands by indebted workers and goods produced in sweatshops by unfree labour. Thus, expropriation supports and amplifies exploitation, embedding it deeply within the capitalist system (Fraser 2023, 14–15).

4   These factors include gender, public or private sector employment, age, marital status, education, tenure, job permanence, full- or part-time status, workplace size, industry, occupation, immigration status, province, census metropolitan area, and unionization (Macdonald 2024, 4).

5   For the latest collection of in-depth analyses on how the capitalist political economy results in unequal health outcomes, refer to Primrose, Loeppky, and Chang (2024). Waitzkin (2024) proposes "creative constructive actions" and "creative destructive actions" to counter capitalism.

CHAPTER SEVEN

Searching for Socialism

If health inequities primarily originate from capitalism, then it is essential to replace this exploitative/oppressive system. Capitalism severely limits social changes and state policies that could better address the needs of people and communities. Instead, we need a societal system and way of life that prioritize the health and well-being of individuals and the environment over profit and wealth accumulation. In the concluding chapters, I explore the fundamentals of socialism, its principles, and how it could improve health equity both within and beyond capitalist frameworks. Socialism offers a hopeful and viable route to achieving health for all.

Welfare Systems in Capitalism

Welfare systems in capitalist states reveal social inequities and health gaps, suggesting various ways to address them. Esping-Andersen (1990) grouped sixteen advanced capitalist countries into three types of welfare systems: liberal, conservative, and social democratic.

In Canada, the US, and Australia, which are *liberal welfare states*, the focus is on using market-based solutions and private-sector services for welfare. This approach exacerbates health gaps, especially for people who cannot afford private services. On the other hand, *conservative welfare states*, like Germany, France, and the Netherlands, rely more on traditional family roles and provide more substantial public services. However, this type makes it difficult for everyone to access health services equally because it reinforces social hierarchies. In contrast, *social democratic welfare states*, such as Sweden, Finland, and Denmark, see the state playing a crucial role in providing robust social support and health services. Regardless of social class, gender, and race, everyone can get the care they need. These socialist-inspired ideas and practices reduce health inequities and improve overall health.

Categorizing welfare states based on factors such as citizenship, rights, de-commodification (treating services as rights, not as commodities), social stratification, and the roles of government, market, and family in social provisioning (Esping-Andersen 1990, 18–26), clearly demonstrates how they impact health outcomes. The welfare state system fundamentally shapes how society functions and how people interact. For instance, social democratic countries provide better pensions and support for people out of work compared to conservative and liberal countries. By studying these different welfare state models, we can gain insights into which systems are more effective at improving health within capitalist frameworks and beyond.

Welfare State Regimes

The liberal welfare state primarily supports lower income, working-class individuals through means-tested programs, limited universal benefits, and basic social insurance. Assistance is selectively provided, targeting those deemed more likely to rely on welfare instead of seeking employment. Consequently, strict eligibility criteria and associated stigma result in minimal support. This system heavily relies on the market and does not offer broad social rights, leading to a society divided into two main groups: one struggling in poverty with minimal government aid, and another whose well-being is closely tied to market performance (Esping-Andersen 1990, 26–27). Overall, this approach emphasizes a small welfare system driven by market forces and traditional work values.

The conservative welfare state differs from the liberal one by focusing on maintaining social hierarchies rather than prioritizing market efficiency and granting rights based on class and status. In this system, the government plays a central role in welfare provision, while private insurance and occupational benefits are less common. Religious institutions, which emphasize traditional family roles, significantly influence this approach. These institutions follow the subsidiarity principle, wherein the government intervenes only when families cannot care for themselves (Esping-Andersen 1990, 27). The conservative welfare state values tradition and social status over the redistribution of wealth and power from capitalists to workers and from elites to the masses.

In social democratic states, everyone receives the same social rights, regardless of social class. This approach provides top-quality services and benefits that even the middle class supports. These countries use a universal insurance system that adjusts benefits based on income levels, thereby reducing the market's role. The goal is to create a more equal society by sharing responsibilities and opportunities. As a result, individuals have more power and less dependence on market pressures or traditional family roles. Instead of relying on families, the state helps care for children, older adults, and those in need. This focus on family-friendly services also allows women to decide if they want to engage in paid employment (Esping-Andersen 1990, 27–29). Social democratic states encourage personal freedom and offer a solid safety net.

In social democratic states, ensuring employment for all is crucial for financial stability. This approach not only promotes societal health but also boosts revenue by increasing workforce participation. Unlike conservative systems, which discourage women from working for wages, and liberal systems, which rely heavily on market forces, social democratic regimes strive to provide equal employment opportunities for women and men (Esping-Andersen 1990, 27–29). This commitment to equality and social welfare is strongly influenced by socialist ideas and practices, which shape the foundation of the social democratic welfare state.

Welfare State Evolution and Influences

Welfare states have evolved due to significant historical shifts, such as the rise of working-class political influence and the transition from predominantly rural societies to more middle-class urban ones. These changes have shaped support for different welfare systems. Historically, state reforms ensured that the middle class supported conservative governments, while in liberal states, the middle class relied more on the private market. Scandinavian countries are unique because they have developed welfare state systems that effectively serve both traditional working-class clientele (blue-collar workers) and white-collar workers (Esping-Andersen 1990, 29–33). The struggles between various social classes, historical events, political movements, and past policy changes have all played significant roles in shaping the formation and functions of welfare states.

Different types of welfare states, such as social democratic, Christian democratic, liberal, and former fascist (as categorized by Navarro and colleagues), illustrate how politics and policies affect health. From 1960 to 1996, social democratic countries had the lowest infant mortality rates compared to other types. In contrast, liberal countries had higher infant mortality rates because powerful capitalists weakened parties and movements that supported the working class (Navarro and Shi 2002). This situation led to fewer state actions to equitably distribute societal wealth, which could have benefited the working class and impoverished people, improved health outcomes, and reduced health inequities.

Countries where social democratic parties and labour movements prioritize everyone's well-being tend to have healthier populations. From 1950 to 1998, governments in OECD countries led by socialist parties promoting equality managed to reduce infant mortality by addressing social inequality (Navarro et al. 2006). This book demonstrates how efforts from the working class and socialist parties in capitalist systems can improve health outcomes and create fairer conditions for all. Achieving health equity through socialism is realizable.

Key Metrics across Welfare State Regimes

In this section, I demonstrate the connections between trade union density, low wages, poverty, and infant mortality. By employing classifications from Navarro and colleagues as well as Esping-Andersen, I analyzed data from OECD countries. Some information is unavailable for specific periods or countries due to missing data (denoted as "n/a"). Nonetheless, the findings underscore commonalities and differences among welfare states, providing insight into the various factors that shape socioeconomic and health outcomes.

Trade Union Density

The percentage of workers in labour unions, known as trade union density, has decreased worldwide over the past few decades. From 1980 to 2020, the average trade union density dropped significantly across various types of welfare states: social democratic (SD) countries saw a decline from about 67% to 54%, Christian democratic (CD) countries from 37% to 23%, liberal Anglo-Saxon (LAS) countries from 43% to 13%, and countries with conservative former fascist dictatorships (CFD) from 44% to 32%. This decline underscores a substantial difference in labour unions' influence, particularly between social democratic and liberal states. The US, a major player in global capitalism, exhibits very low levels of union presence.

TABLE 7.1 TRADE UNION DENSITY

	1960 %	1970 %	1980 %	1990 %	2000 %	2010 %	2020 %
OECD AVERAGE	38.0	37.9	36.5	28.8	20.9	17.8	15.8 (2019)
Social Democratic							
Austria	60.1	56.7	51.7	46.8	36.9	28.9	26.3 (2019)
Denmark	59.0	60.8	77.2	73.9	74.5	68.1	67.0 (2019)
Finland	31.9	51.3	69.4	72.6	74.2	71.4	58.8
Norway	60.0	56.8	57.9	58.5	53.6	50.5	50.4 (2019)
Sweden	64.6	66.6	78.1	81.5	81.0	68.2	65.2 (2019)
SD AVERAGE	55.1	58.4	66.9	66.7	64.0	57.4	53.4
Christian Democratic							
Belgium	41.5	42.1	53.4	50.6	56.6	53.0	49.1 (2019)
France	20.0	22.1	18.6	10.7	10.8	10.8	10.8 (2016)
Germany	34.7	32.1	34.9	31.2	24.6	18.9	16.3 (2019)
Italy	28.5	36.3	49.6	39.0	34.8	35.3	32.5 (2019)
Netherlands	41.7	38.1	34.8	24.6	22.3	19.5	15.4 (2019)
Switzerland	31.2	25.4	28.1	23.0	20.7	17.6	14.4 (2018)
CD AVERAGE	32.9	32.7	36.6	29.9	28.3	25.6	23.1
Liberal Anglo-Saxon							
Australia	53.8	44.2	49.6	41.3	24.9	18.4	13.7 (2018)
Canada	30.1	31.8	34.0	33.6	28.2	27.2	27.2
Ireland	45.3	53.2	57.1	51.1	35.9	31.6	26.2
United Kingdom	40.5	44.8	52.2	39.6	29.8	26.6	23.5 (2019)
United States	30.9	27.4	22.1	15.5	12.9	11.4	10.3
LAS AVERAGE	40.1	40.3	43.0	36.2	26.3	23.0	12.7
Conservative Former Fascist Dictatorship							
Greece	n/a	48.2 (1977)	39.0	35.2 (1989)	24.9 (2001)	22.2	19.0 (2016)
Portugal	n/a	70.5 (1973)	78.1	81.5	81.0	68.2	65.2 (2019)
Spain	n/a	18.1 (1977)	13.3	14.1	17.5	18.2	12.5 (2019)
CFD AVERAGE	n/a	45.6	43.5	43.6	41.1	36.2	32.2

Note: The figures represent the percentage of workers who are in labour unions. Source: OECD (2024a).

The global decline in union membership worldwide signifies the growing influence of neoliberalism. This trend indicates that capitalists and policymakers favouring capitalism are gaining strength while socialist and labour movements are losing their foothold in societal affairs. Strong unions have historically supported workers, yet many people may not recognize that capitalism is the root cause of social and health problems. Consequently, there is often a lack of awareness about the necessity to move beyond capitalism for an improved quality of life.

Low-Wage Rates

This section investigates the relationship between trade union density and wage levels from 2000 to 2020. Wages are categorized into low and high pay, with low-paid workers earning below two-thirds of the median and high-paid workers earning more than 1.5 times the median (OECD 2024b). The data, expressed in percentages, focuses on full-time employees.

Analyzing low-wage trends across different welfare states reveals notable differences. Conservative former fascist dictatorships show the lowest average low-pay rates, slightly outperforming Christian democratic and social democratic states by 2020. For example, with a high trade union density of 65.2%, Portugal maintains a low-wage rate of 5.3%, indicating that greater union density can lead to better wages. However, this positive correlation is inconsistent; Italy, with a moderate trade union density of 32.5%, reports the lowest low-wage rate at 3.6%, suggesting that factors beyond trade union density influence wage levels. See Table 2.

Such inconsistencies are typical in welfare state comparisons. Although social democratic countries do not always yield the best results, a trend is evident: lower union density is generally associated with higher low-pay rates, particularly in liberal welfare states. For instance, the US, with the lowest trade union density at 10.3%, has the highest low-pay rate at 23.8% in 2020. A capitalist powerhouse, the US does not provide the most favourable environment for most workers.

Poverty Rates

This section examines the influence of trade union density and low pay on poverty rates. The poverty rate measures the proportion of the population earning less than the established poverty threshold, defined as 50% of the median income for households across the population. This metric is available by age group: children (0-17 years), working-age adults (18-65), and older adults (66 years and above). Table 7.3 shows the poverty rate

TABLE 7.2 LOW-WAGE RATES

	2000–05 %	2010 %	2020 %
OECD AVERAGE	**16.7**	**15.4**	**14.1**
Social Democratic			
Austria	n/a	16.5	14.7
Denmark	7.4 (2002)	7.6	9.5 (2021)
Finland	4.6 (2001)	8.1	8.4 (2021)
Norway	n/a	n/a	n/a
Sweden	n/a	n/a	n/a
SD AVERAGE	**6.0**	**10.7**	**10.9**
Christian Democratic			
Belgium	6.3 (2004)	4.3	12
France	7.2 (2002)	5.8	5.3
Germany	15.7	19.0	17.0
Italy	5.7 (2002)	8.1	3.6
Netherlands	9.6 (2002)	7.9	6.0
Switzerland	n/a	13.1	12.0
CD AVERAGE	**8.9**	**9.7**	**9.3**
Liberal Anglo-Saxon			
Australia	16.4	16.4	15.5 (2019)
Canada	23.3	21.2	18.7
Ireland	16.5 (2002)	17.7	18.0 (2019)
United Kingdom	20.9	20.7	18.0
United States	24.7	25.3	23.8
LAS AVERAGE	**20.4**	**20.3**	**18.8**
Conservative Former Fascist Dictatorship			
Greece	12.3 (2002)	12.6	12.1
Portugal	17.3 (2002)	15.9	5.3
Spain	13.3 (2002)	10.6	8.9
CFD AVERAGE	**14.3**	**13.0**	**8.8**

Note: the figures represent the percentage of full-time employees who are in low-wage employment.
Source: OECD (2024b).

TABLE 7.3 POVERTY RATES

	2000-2005 %	2010-2015 %	2020 %
Social Democratic			
Austria	n/a	8.9	9.6
Denmark	n/a	5.8 (2011)	6.5 (2019)
Finland	5.3	7.2	5.7
Norway	6.9 (2004)	7.5	8.4
Sweden	n/a	8.4 (2013)	8.8
SD AVERAGE	6.1	7.56	7.8
Christian Democratic			
Belgium	n/a	n/a	7.3
France	n/a	n/a	7.7
Germany	n/a	8.7 (2011)	11.6
Italy	12.2 (2004)	13.4	13.5
Netherlands	n/a	7.2 (2011)	8.2
Switzerland	n/a	9.4	9.9
CD AVERAGE	n/a	9.675	9.7
Liberal Anglo-Saxon			
Australia	n/a	14 (2012)	12.6
Canada	12	13.1	8.6
Ireland	13.4 (2004)	9.1	7.7
United Kingdom	12.6 (2002)	11	11.2
United States	n/a	17.2 (2013)	16.4
LAS AVERAGE	12.67	12.88	11.3
Conservative Fascist Dictatorship			
Greece	12 (2004)	14.1	13
Portugal	13.2 (2004)	10.9	12.8
Spain	n/a	13.9	15.4
CFD AVERAGE	12.6	12.97	13.73

Source: OECD (2024c).

as a percentage of the population. It is important to note that even if two countries share similar poverty rates, the relative incomes of their impoverished populations might differ (OECD 2024c). Our analysis covers the period from 2000 to 2020, providing insights into the evolving relationship between trade union density, low pay, and poverty across demographics.

Since the 2000s, social democratic countries have seen a rise in poverty, except Finland, where it declined to 5.7% in 2020. Despite this trend, social democratic countries still maintain the lowest average poverty rates across different welfare regimes. Christian democratic countries have experienced relatively stable poverty rates, except for Germany, which has seen a significant increase, and Italy, which peaked at 13.5% in 2020. Conversely, the conservative former fascist dictatorships have experienced a rise in average poverty rates since the 2000s, with Spain leading at 15.4% in 2020.

In 2020, the poverty level in liberal Anglo-Saxon countries dropped to 11.3%, driven by significant decreases in Canada (down to 8.6%) and Ireland's (down to 7.7%) from 2010 to 2020. The US, however, had the highest poverty rate among these countries at 16.4% in 2020. This suggests that in the US, lower trade union density is strongly associated with lower pay rates and, consequently, higher poverty rates.

Infant Mortality Rates

Trade union membership, low wages, and poverty rates significantly impact infant mortality rates, which are the number of deaths in the first year of life per 1000 live births. As previously mentioned, poverty — often resulting from low wages and income — disproportionately affects certain groups: women, people of colour, older adults, young people, 2SLGBTQIA+ individuals, and people with disabilities. While poverty undeniably affects health, the root cause of health inequities lies in the capitalist system. Capitalism not only generates poverty but also exacerbates health problems. The correlation between increased poverty and rising infant mortality rates illustrates how capitalist systems fundamentally shape unequal socioeconomic and health outcomes.

Infant mortality rates have consistently declined across various welfare state regimes since the 1960s. By 2020, liberal Anglo-Saxon countries had the highest infant mortality rates, followed by Christian democratic, conservative former fascist dictatorships, and social democratic countries. It is important to note that the registration practices for premature infants can affect comparisons. For instance, the US and Canada register more infants weighing below 500 grams, leading to higher reported infant mortality rates. In contrast, some European countries use criteria like a gestational age of 22 weeks or a 500 gram birth weight to count live births (OECD 2024d). Even adjusting for these factors, liberal Anglo-Saxon countries still likely rank highest in infant mortality rates. Furthermore, while Canada's infant mortality rate has dropped significantly, stark disparities persist between its richest and poorest populations, highlighting ongoing health inequities.

TABLE 7.4 INFANT MORTALITY RATES

	1960 %	1970 %	1980 %	1990 %	2000 %	2010 %	2020 %
OECD							
Social Democratic							
Austria	37.5	25.9	14.3	7.8	4.8	3.9	3.1
Denmark	21.5	14.2	8.4	7.5	5.3	3.3	2.4
Finland	21.0	13.2	7.6	5.6	3.8	2.3	1.8
Norway	16.0	12.8	8.3	6.9	3.9	2.5	1.6
Sweden	16.6	11.0	6.9	6.0	3.4	2.5	2.4
SD AVERAGE	**22.5**	**15.42**	**9.1**	**6.76**	**4.24**	**2.9**	**2.3**
Christian Democratic							
Belgium	31.4	21.1	12.1	8.0	4.8	3.6	3.3
France	27.7	18.2	10.0	7.3	4.5	3.6	3.6
Germany	33.8	23.6	12.6	7.0	4.4	3.4	3.1
Italy	43.9	29.6	14.6	8.1	4.3	3.0	2.4
Netherlands	16.5	12.7	8.6	7.1	5.1	3.8	3.8
Switzerland	21.1	15.1	9.1	6.8	4.9	3.8	3.6
CD AVERAGE	**29.01**	**20.05**	**11.12**	**7.38**	**4.67**	**3.53**	**3.3**
Liberal Anglo-Saxon							
Australia	20.2	17.9	10.7	8.2	5.2	4.1	3.2
Canada	27.3	18.8	10.4	6.8	5.3	5.0	4.5
Ireland	29.3	19.5	11.1	8.2	6.2	3.6	3.0
United Kingdom	22.5	18.5	12.1	7.9	5.6	4.2	3.8
United States	26.0	20.0	12.6	9.2	6.9	6.1	5.4
LAS AVERAGE	**25.1**	**18.9**	**12.9**	**8.06**	**5.84**	**6.1**	**4.0**
Conservative Fascist Dictatorship							
Greece	40.1	29.6	17.9	9.7	5.9	3.8	3.2
Portugal	77.5	55.5	24.3	10.9	5.5	2.5	2.4
Spain	43.7	28.1	12.3	7.6	4.4	3.2	2.6
CFD AVERAGE	**53.8**	**37.7**	**18.2**	**9.4**	**5.3**	**3.2**	**2.7**

Note: The figures represent the number of deaths in the first year of life per 1000 live births.
Source: OECD (2024d).

TABLE 7.5 TRADE UNION DENSITY, LOW-WAGE RATES, POVERTY RATES, AND INFANT MORTALITY RATES

	Trade Union Density %		Low-Wage Rate %		Poverty Rate %		Infant Mortality Rate %	
AVERAGE	2000	2020	2000	2020	2000	2020	2000	2020
SD	64	53.4	6.0	10.9	6.1	7.8	4.24	2.3
CD	28.3	23.1	8.9	9.3	n/a	9.7	4.67	3.3
LAS	26.3	12.7	20.4	18.8	12.67	11.3	5.84	4.0
CFD	41.1	32.2	14.3	8.8	10.6	13.4	5.3	2.7

Tables 7.1–7.5 illustrate the connections between trade union density, low wages, poverty, and infant mortality. Table 7.5 highlights that liberal welfare states consistently have the lowest trade union membership and the highest rates of low wages, poverty, and infant mortality. The US Empire, in particular, shows poor outcomes in these areas. This trend suggests that lower union density is associated with increased issues such as low pay, poverty, and infant deaths. The data implies that the capitalist system fails to improve living conditions for many, indicating that socialism may offer a more beneficial alternative for achieving better societal outcomes.

Lessons from Welfare State Regimes and Neoliberalism

In liberal welfare regimes, state policies favouring big businesses harm workers and ordinary people. These policies benefit the capitalists and the wealthy, leaving many without enough resources such as jobs, income, housing, and health care. To improve individual, family, and population health, we need socialist policies and social actions that address these issues.

The Role of Social Democracy

Capitalist countries, particularly those in the liberal Anglo-Saxon group, face significant challenges with working conditions and public health. In contrast, countries with social democratic systems, which incorporate socialist principles, generally achieve better health outcomes. This trend suggests that socialist policies, supported by strong labour movements and socialist political parties, can influence state decisions to benefit everyone.

However, it is important to note that social democracy — while incorporating some socialist ideas and practices, such as wealth and power redistribution — still supports capitalism (Clarke 2021). This reality presents a significant problem for genuine socialist parties and movements. Social democracy aims to reform capitalism but yields to capitalist pressures, undermining efforts to overcome capitalism and liberate workers and the masses from its control. Contemporary social democracy increasingly embraces capitalist policies due to class divisions and the influence of capital interests on state decisions. Even in countries with robust social programs, capitalism maintains a strong influence. This ongoing struggle between the desire for social justice and the power of capitalism makes achieving health equity within a capitalist framework challenging.

The Role of Trade Unions

When trade unions are not strong and united, they can exacerbate social and health inequities. Union leaders and organizers encounter significant roadblocks in unifying workers from diverse backgrounds and with varying issues, such as those facing additional challenges due to race, ethnicity, or gender (Borras 2021, 2022, 2023). Additionally, many contemporary trade unions do not openly oppose capitalism or advocate for socialism.

Workers' situations worsen partly because trade unions do not adequately educate members about the connections between health, work, politics, and economics. Union representatives often fail to explain how capitalism impacts workers and why they should oppose it. This lack of awareness makes it difficult for workers to identify capitalism as the main problem and view socialism as a viable solution to improve their lives. Furthermore, many low-income workers are preoccupied with day-to-day survival, leaving them with little time to engage in union activities and politics. This weak connection between union officials and members allows capitalism to dominate social life.

Many trade unions today primarily act as go-betweens for workers and bosses. They have evolved into large bureaucracies with limited democratic processes, where only a few individuals, mainly top officials, have a say in decision making (Evans et al. 2023). This corporate-like structure raises doubts about their willingness to challenge capitalism as an adversary. As more workers and people advocate for societal change through socialism (Thompson 2023), it becomes evident that traditional trade unions are unlikely to lead this transformation or revolutionize society. Therefore, workers must establish new ways to drive real change — a socialist union and movement that opposes the capitalist way of life.

We need a fresh workers' movement that challenges capitalism and supports socialism. Socialist workers, community movements, and political parties from all levels should unite to achieve *Socialism for All*. This broad coalition of socialist forces must struggle against capitalism and for socialism to improve the environment, society, and people's lives.

We must recognize that social democracy, trade unions, and even some socialists have not fully demonstrated how capitalism affects different groups of workers, exacerbating divisions. To address this confusion, socialists must empower the working class and establish a robust socialist party. This party would aim to break the ties between Big Capital and state apparatuses. By promoting socialist ideas and practices in workplaces, communities, and governments, we can challenge the dominance of capitalism and transform societal structures.

The Role of Socialists

In the fight against capitalism and for socialism, many socialists become entangled in prolonged theoretical debates on the best ways to achieve socialism. These higher level but often abstract discussions may emphasize the importance of a vanguard party, the need for a working-class revolution, and the supporting roles of peasants and other people's movements. While these debates are necessary, they can sometimes become redundant and distract from actual practical actions and the essential truth that real transformative power lies with the masses, who have historically been the decisive agents of societal revolution. Although the working class should be at the forefront of the class struggle, the supreme power belongs to the masses — the people.

While social democratic parties, like Canada's New Democratic Party, might advocate for changes and socialist ideas, they act like traditional parties. For example, instead of fostering critical dialogue, they expel those who disagree with top leadership (Beattie and Hristova 2023). Such actions demonstrate that social democrats lack confidence in the ability of workers and ordinary people to make crucial decisions for society. Unlike social democrats, genuine socialists steadfastly believe in the abilities of ordinary people. They work to enhance and harness these capacities, empowering them to take control of the means of production, the state, and its apparatuses. Their goal is to meet public needs (Marx and Engels [1848] 1964), rather than the private desires of economic and political elites. This stance underscores a firm conviction in the transformative potential of collective worker action and the critical role of the masses in building a fair and healthier society.

Some socialists argue antagonistically against different socialist ideas and practices, which is counterproductive. It is essential to recognize that socialism is a dynamic process, not a static ideology. As an alternative system to capitalism, it must continually adapt and innovate to fit new concrete situations. Therefore, instead of engaging in divisive internal conflicts, socialists should collaborate to enhance socialist theories and practices for the benefit of all. Seeing socialism as an ongoing process means understanding that it always has room to grow. Instead of sticking to just one way of thinking, we should welcome different socialist ideas and practices as opportunities for improvement. This flexible, non-dogmatic stance encourages trying new approaches and learning from them to improve socialism. By being open to change, socialists can foster collaborative endeavours and be more effective against capitalist forces.

Establishing socialism requires a good balance of practical action and theoretical discussion. We must continuously educate, organize, and rally workers and the masses for real societal change. While theories are important, the priority should be on practices that resonate with people's everyday lives and aspirations. Socialism advances when it adapts to real-life challenges. Viewing socialism as a complex adaptive system emphasizes the importance of informed social activism and political actions. This perspective is crucial for empowering the oppressed and exploited, providing them tools to understand capitalism and to find ways to emancipate themselves through socialism. Socialism is not just a theory but a practice that improves human societies. By making socialism practical and flexible, we can transform it into a powerful movement for health equity.

Pathways to Addressing Health Inequities

The big questions in addressing health inequities are: What should we do differently, and how do we do it? We need to learn from both past and present experiences. Edwin Chadwick (1842) suggested reformist policy changes within capitalism, while Karl Marx and Friedrich Engels ([1848] 1964) advocated for a revolutionary social change. They argued that a class revolution is necessary to overthrow and replace capitalism with socialism or communism to achieve true equality and fairness.

Today, it is widely recognized that improving health requires addressing how social class, gender, and race are connected. For instance, political economist and health policy expert Vicente Navarro (2020), working in the tradition of Marx and Engels, emphasizes the need for an emancipatory project to end all forms of oppression, including those based on class, gender, race, nationality, and environmental exploitation. We must recognize these connections as part of a broader effort against capitalism. Our goal should be to replace capitalism with a system that fosters harmony between human beings and nature. This new system should be a fair, equal, and eco-friendly socialist system that opposes exploitation and oppression.

In the battle against capitalism, we need a strategy that balances leadership with active listening and involvement. It is crucial to understand people's situations and value their experiences. Instead of just following leaders or only considering members' perspectives, we should encourage open conversations and learn from each other. This collaborative approach allows everyone to shape our path toward socialism and health equity. It is a long journey, but by working together against exploitation and oppression in all forms, we can build healthy societies.

Challenging and Overcoming Capitalism

Erik Olin Wright's (2015, 2018) analysis of anti-capitalist movements offers different ways to challenge or move beyond capitalism. He outlines six strategies: smashing, dismantling, taming, resisting, escaping, and eroding capitalism. Each strategy has its reasons, methods, and plausible results. How could these strategies apply in today's world?

1. *Smashing capitalism.* Some believe in a revolutionary strategy to end capitalism, which involves overthrowing the system entirely. Proponents argue that capitalism is deeply flawed and leads to recurring crises. By seizing the state through revolutions or elections, they aim to replace capitalism with socialism, where resources are owned by everyone and shared equally. While past revolutions have faced obstacles, they are seen as essential steps in moving away from capitalism. Supporters believe we can learn from past failures to create a fairer society by significantly changing our economy (Wright 2015, 2018). This strategy fights for a radical transformation of the economic system to achieve a more equitable distribution of resources.

2. *Dismantling capitalism.* Another approach is democratic socialism, which slowly changes capitalism by adding socialist ideas. This means using state reforms to create a mix of capitalism and

socialism, aiming for a better economy. It involves a socialist political party working within the current system to introduce policies that reduce inequities. Unlike revolutionary change, democratic socialism prefers steady progress instead of sudden change. It is not easy because it faces resistance from those who want to preserve the way things are. Revolutionary and gradual approaches aim to replace capitalism with socialism but take different paths (Wright 2015, 2018).

3. *Taming capitalism.* Taming capitalism aims to mitigate its negative impacts through state policies. This strategy advocates for better pay, job security, and workplace safety. It also supports policies to reduce inequality and protect the environment. While this approach does not tackle the root problems of capitalism, it lessens its adverse effects, akin to treating symptoms without curing the underlying illness. In the past, this was done by social democratic parties that wanted gradual changes rather than revolutions. It worked well for a while, with policies like social insurance and better wages (Wright 2015, 2018), but recent changes have made capitalism more harmful and dangerous. This strategy focuses on incremental reforms without addressing the fundamental issues inherent in the capitalist system.

4. *Resisting capitalism.* Resisting capitalism fights against its harmful effects without taking over the state and its apparatuses. People use protests and other actions to pressure businesses and politicians to do better. This approach is popular among grassroots organizations like environmentalist groups and unions fighting for workers' rights. These efforts often connect with issues like race and gender equality. Groups like trade unions use strikes and negotiations to improve conditions at work. This resistance occurs in workplaces and the streets, even when the ruling government is not supportive (Wright 2015, 2018). This strategy leverages grassroots activism and direct action to challenge capitalism's negative impacts and advocate for social justice without seeking state power.

5. *Escaping capitalism.* Escaping capitalism involves finding ways to live apart from its influence. Some people believe capitalism is too entrenched to change, so they live independently. This strategy can include starting farms or communes or living simpler

lives away from the pressures of money and competition. Groups like the Amish have been doing this for generations. Others opt for early retirement and live off savings instead of working for big companies. While this approach is more individualistic than collective and not applicable for everyone (Wright 2015, 2018), it demonstrates alternative living beyond the reach of capitalism. This strategy explores ways to live self-reliantly, showcasing diverse approaches to escaping capitalism's constraints.

6. *Eroding capitalism.* Eroding capitalism is a unique way of challenging it by creating alternative systems within the capitalist framework. This strategy involves mixing businesses with cooperatives and community networks to reduce capitalism's control gradually. It is like planting seeds of change within the current system. Inspired by modern anarchism, this approach differs from more revolutionary or reformist strategies. It tries to create small-scale alternatives that can grow over time, similar to how capitalism replaced feudalism. This approach blends grassroots movements with state-centric strategies, as seen in Syriza and Podemos, which aim to diminish capitalism's influence by promoting democratic and cooperative practices. While offering an alternative path, it faces corporate pushback, particularly in environments where the government is unsupportive (Wright 2015, 2018). This strategy seeks to undermine capitalism's dominance by fostering democratic economic models within the existing system.

Wright (2015, 2018) ultimately suggests a multi-pronged approach against capitalism. It involves a mix of dismantling, taming, resisting, and escaping capitalism's influence. This approach includes state actions to reduce the adverse effects of capitalism and support more empowering economic activities. It relies on collective resistance from labour unions, community organizations, and social movements, aiming to uphold democracy, equality, and solidarity. To move beyond capitalism, a diverse strategy is essential. This strategy encompasses directly challenging capitalism, transforming it from within, establishing rules to control its power, engaging in militant activism, and creating socialist alternatives for a better society. As capitalism evolves, advocates of true socialism must adapt and innovate new solutions to contemporary challenges, recognizing that socialism offers a different way of organizing society. Socialism heralds a different world order. We must chart a new course toward socialism and equitable health for all.

Circling and Countering Capitalism for Health Equity

Improving health fairness requires examining how institutions, cultures, politics, and economics affect health and health care. Our health politics must challenge the alliance of capital and state. We must combine various anti-capitalism strategies to advance socialism and health equity.

Paths toward Health Equity

As health inequities worsen, there is an opportunity for meaningful change, that is, moving away from capitalism and toward socialism. First, overthrowing capitalism to achieve health equity could occur through protests and other actions beyond voting. Second, engaging in health politics and policymaking is vital as it sets the stage for breaking capitalism and achieving health equity. Initiating this process opens the door toward democratic socialism, which can substantially reduce health inequities. Third, while pushing for health equity policies curbs capitalism's harm, social democracy — with its mix of capitalist and socialist ideas — has an inherent flaw. It underestimates the power of everyday people to bring about change. Social democrats think they have all the answers to address health inequities instead of listening to diverse views. The real challenge is uniting different groups, especially grassroots socialist movements and political parties. This unity is central to gaining the power needed to achieve health for all. Fourth, in the quest for health equity, many labour unions, community organizations, and social movements repel capitalism. However, this strategy operates autonomously from the state and seeks no direct governmental control to address health inequities. Fifth, distancing from political engagement to evade the pitfalls of capitalism safeguards individual well-being. However, this is a romantic rather than realistic approach to health equity, as one cannot truly avoid the tentacles of capitalism. Lastly, a health equity approach that seeks to corrode capital dominance gradually combines top-down government initiatives to curb and break capitalism with bottom-up actions designed to evade and repel it.

Corroding capitalism presents a promising avenue for addressing health inequities. Take Newfoundland and Labrador as an example. The provincial government teamed up with grassroots community groups to fight poverty, implementing policies like making housing more affordable, giving people money back on taxes, freezing tuition fees, assisting with childcare, and pumping more money into health care. Because of these efforts, fewer people live in poverty there. This *sandwich strategy* shows that combining big government and local community actions can make a real difference. However, whether the state creates changes or people push for them, sufficient and sustained bottom-up pressure is necessary to make socialist-oriented policies a reality (Borras 2016, 57–59).[1] This example illustrates the power of combined state and societal efforts to effectively address poverty, a critical factor in health inequities.

Electoral Politics

Exercising caution is wise when participating in electoral politics to shape health policies. The alliance between capital and the state actors significantly influences this arena. With their combined wealth and power, compared to socialist forces, capitalist forces maintain sustained political governance, as demonstrated by the history of ruling federal governments in Canada. Consequently, socialism cannot truly emerge through the current parliamentary system because it vigorously protects and supports capitalism. As Audre Lorde (2018) said, "The master's tools will never dismantle the master's house." The capitalist state will never commit political suicide by instituting electoral reforms that will weaken its political power. Nevertheless, recent changes in global politics show a rise in the support for socialist-leaning political leaders and parties. In the US, the Squad is becoming more influential. Brazil's Lula da Silva, Bolivia's Evo Morales and Luis Arce, and Chile's Gabriel Boric have come to power, indicating increasing support for socialist ideas and policies. Union leader Leody de Guzman, academic activist Walden Bello, and labour lawyer Luke Espiritu openly challenged the wealthy families and political dynasties in the Philippines. Although not expected to win, their political campaigns have raised awareness about socialism.

In July 2024, the New Popular Front in France won the most seats in the National Assembly, while the Labour Party ended Conservative rule in the UK general election. These victories signal a shift in public sentiment, reflecting the aspirations of workers and the broader population to move away from neoliberal policies and counter the rise of far-right movements. Both election outcomes indicate a desire for change and a renewed focus on social and economic justice. Left-leaning individuals and groups must inform and educate the public about how money influences state policies and elections, emphasizing the need to unite the working classes and popular movements to challenge the entrenched capital-state alliance at municipal, provincial, national, and global levels.

Elections serve as a way to examine who holds wealth and power and how they use it. They are critical because they expose what is wrong with our system and how capitalism harms the people and the environment. They also allow us to educate, organize, and rally against societal and health problems. When ordinary people get involved, they can push politicians to listen and improve the working, living, and health conditions for everyone. Thus, the forces of socialism must empower people toward massive decentralization and democratization of politics and the economy for its establishment.

Further Reflection

Social democracy — a softer version of capitalism — makes minor improvements but remains part of the capitalist system. While social democracy can slowly chip away at capitalism, genuine socialists aim to replace it with socialism. The key to achieving this is harnessing the power of regular people. Real change transpires when people unite and decide they have had enough of capitalism's flaws and harms. Ultimately, it is up to us to push for a better societal system.

The critical political economy approach to health inequities examines capital, labour, civil society, and state relations. Marx and Engels emphasized the role of economic relations and class struggle, particularly between the capitalist and working classes, as the main drivers of social change and human development. They argued that the state primarily serves as an extension of the power of the capitalist class (Engels 1845; Marx and Engels [1848] 1964; Marx 1867). After Marx and Engels, Antonio Gramsci and Nicos Poulantzas enriched the Marxist understanding of the state.

Gramsci (1971) contended that the ruling class increasingly employs cultural structures, such as education and media, to secure consent from civil society (e.g., trade union concessions) and maintain legitimacy. However, coercion remains a tool the state utilizes to uphold capital power, particularly in times of threat. Poulantzas (2020) further argued that the state organizes the capitalist classes, maintaining an "unstable equilibrium of compromise" with the working classes and other subordinated groups. However, despite its relative autonomy, the state remains a stronghold of Big Capital, forming a strategic alliance favouring capital accumulation at the expense of the working class and public interests. Understanding this fundamental notion about the state is crucial for comprehending the actions and inactions of the contemporary capitalist state on health inequities.

The alternative road, genuine socialism, envisions a world where workers and community members collectively own ecological resources and societal wealth. If socialism aims to address all the injustices of capitalism, it faces an enormous challenge. It must create a new societal order that transcends not only class domination but also gender and sex inequalities, neocolonial and imperial-racial-ethnic oppression, and political domination in all forms. Additionally, it must deinstitutionalize entrenched crisis tendencies, including economic, financial, ecological, social-reproductive, and political. Socialism for today's world must also significantly expand the range of democracy — not merely by democratizing decision making within a pre-existing political framework but by redefining and reshaping the boundaries and concepts that constitute "the political" (Fraser 2023, 151). Socialist theories and practices must undergo ongoing iterative processes to attain their full potential. Socialism is achievable when socialists are open, flexible, and adaptive to ever-changing concrete material and social conditions of life.

The new socialist vision advocates for communal ownership originating from the grassroots, not imposed by the state bureaucrats but built from the ground up by workers and the masses. It embodies grassroots socialism, powered and steered by a diverse coalition of socialists, workers, and individuals committed to informing, educating, advocating, organizing, and mobilizing against capitalist forces within and outside the state (Borras 2022). These open, articulate, and dedicated socialists stand united, tactically and strategically, in opposing capitalism and supporting socialism. This collective endeavour marks a transformative journey toward a genuinely socialist society en route to health equity.

Note

1   For a detailed exploration of state-society interactions and the sandwich strategy approach, refer to Fox (1993).

CHAPTER EIGHT

Mobilizing for Health Equity

The existence and persistence of health inequities is fundamentally due to capitalism, which generates many social and health problems. By informing, educating, advocating, organizing, and mobilizing for social justice and health equity, we can move away from capitalism, which harms both people and the planet. Mobilizing to achieve health equity requires workers, scholars, activists, and those concerned with social issues to understand socialism and struggle for socialist policies within and beyond capitalism. Health activism toward socialism is essential; the road to health equity is socialism.

The Essence of Socialism

Socialism offers an alternative way to organize society. Unlike capitalism, which focuses on profit maximization and wealth accumulation, socialism emphasizes caring for nature and people's health. It is not merely a modification of capitalism but a fundamentally different system with distinct ideas and goals (Wood 1995, 162). Rather than focusing on individual success, socialism advocates for collective efforts toward ecological, societal, and human development.

In the capitalist system, the capitalists own the means of production, such as factories and land. In this system, the workers contribute more labour than they are paid for, and capitalists earn huge profits from this surplus labour. In contrast, socialism envisions the public, community, or state (albeit a radically restructured state) owning the means of production. Work is organized collectively, and workers equitably share the rewards of their labour. The economy is planned to meet the community's needs rather than making profits for a few people (Marx and Engels [1848] 1964). Socialism builds a world where people collaborate for the common good instead of competing for personal gain, aiming to establish a sustainable way of life for all. Socialist societies aim to make the necessities of life — such as housing, health care, education, utilities, transportation, energy, banks, and natural resources — owned and managed by the people, community, and state. These sectors are vital for the environment and people's well-being. By eliminating the profit motive, socialist societies ensure these services are available to all, not just those who can afford them.

Creating a genuinely socialist state means changing the current organizational structures. Instead of the usual top-down method where state decisions come from a few people at the top, we need a grassroots, bottom-up approach that directly involves the masses. This means ordinary people, not just the leaders, have a voice in governing our society. By doing so, the state can adhere to the main principles of socialism, such as the equal sharing of power and resources to improve the environment, society, and people's lives.

Socialist Processes toward Economic and Social Transformation

In a socialist society, individuals collaboratively work with shared resources, directing their diverse skills and efforts as a unified workforce. This community of workers decides what needs fulfilling and orchestrates their varied labour in an organized manner. Planning is rooted in a collective understanding that all members are part of an interconnected, extensive social system. Individuals join forces to use resources for the benefit of all. Communities work together to produce, share, use, and replenish resources, always striving for the common good. This unified effort ensures that society operates smoothly and fairly (Lebowitz 2023). The economy serves the people and community, resulting in a balanced and just society.

People first identify their needs and capabilities through local groups in a socialist society. These groups include community councils, which track the needs of people and their surroundings, and workers' councils, which directly fulfill those needs. Information about these needs and abilities is then shared with larger assemblies, which prioritize what is most important for society. Individuals and workers from all levels are involved in these decisions. Based on these collective decisions, society plans to use its labour to meet current and future needs. Thus, the community's needs and long-term plans guide how work is assigned (Lebowitz 2023). In socialism, information flows from the bottom-up, guiding top-down decisions to ensure that society's resources are used to benefit everyone. Socialist societies believe in real democracy and working together to plan for the future.

At the core of socialism is the principle that all should have the chance to reach their full potential and thrive in all aspects of life. This conviction, inspired by Marx, aims to create well-rounded individuals. This vision is essential and cannot be compromised, as it clashes with existing social and health inequities. Following Marx and Engels' idea that "the free development of each is the condition for the free development of all," socialism aims to distribute work fairly to resolve imbalances inherited from past systems (Lebowitz 2023). Socialist societies promote the growth of every person to improve overall prosperity. Thus, collective well-being becomes everyone's wealth and health.

In building a socialist society, planning together as a community is crucial. This process goes beyond just making plans; it also changes people and how they relate to each other. Taking part in such revolutionary practice has two results: it changes situations and transforms the people involved. In socialist groups, the time and effort spent making decisions together are not just about finding answers; they also help people learn, grow, and develop bonds, strengthening local, national, and global solidarity (Lebowitz 2023). Building socialism from the ground-up is a promising way to fight social inequalities and improve the health of individuals, families, and communities. Socialism offers a system that can better tackle health inequities than the current one. Our urgent task is building socialism.

Health Activism toward Socialism

I propose helping to establish socialism through health activism. This endeavour involves interlinking methods such as discussing health problems, spreading knowledge, collaborating with others, and advocating policy changes that benefit the workers and masses instead of the capitalists and elites. As health activists, we must develop people's capacities, fight for what is just, and strive towards socialism to improve working and living conditions and address health inequities. Governments and professional organizations mandate that health care workers, such as nurses and personal support workers, participate in advocacy for safeguarding public health. Thus, we must push for new rules that ensure everyone stays healthy.

Some local public health units champion health equity to fill a perceived gap in effective policy action on the social determinants of health by those in power (Raphael and Sayani 2019). However, despite community health centres improving health care access and addressing the social determinants of health, significant challenges block their influence on public policy. These challenges include a lack of resources, conflicting priorities, the limitations of non-profit status, and financial constraints (Cheff 2017). Advocacy alone is insufficient to bridge health gaps.

While public health advocacy addresses the social causes of health inequities, a significant gap exists in translating these ideals into widespread practice. One major obstacle is the emphasis on personal responsibility for health choices, which mirrors a neoliberal mindset prioritizing individual and market-driven solutions to health issues (Cohen and Marshall 2017, 321-22). The health sector must confront these challenges at several levels. It is essential to address the role of business and state policies in perpetuating health inequities. Mobilizing the workforce and health activists is vital, as their collective action is pivotal in achieving health equity.

Understanding how workers and communities participate in health activism — through advocacy, mobilizing, and organizing — is imperative. Advocacy is the most basic level of involvement. It relies on professionals, limiting engagement from the general public. Mobilizing goes a step further by involving larger groups. However, it usually depends on those already actively involved, with staff leading rather than empowering the workforce and community. In both methods, professionals, rather than everyday people, are viewed as the primary agents of change (Gindin 2023; McAlevey 2016). It is crucial to engage a broader range of people, not just professional activists, to realize socialism through health activism.

Organizing brings people together, including those previously uninvolved and unorganized. Here, the power lies with regular folks — the masses — who understand power dynamics, plan tactics and strategies, and achieve goals. They are central in driving economic and social transformation (Gindin 2023; McAlevey 2016). Through organizing, those most impacted, like workers and people living in poverty, take the lead, ensuring that social justice and health equity struggles are genuinely participatory, democratic, and liberating.

Health activism for socialism requires ongoing united efforts from individuals and people's movements. Socialism through health activism means working to build a society where the needs of workers and communities come before those of wealthy capitalists. As the world deals with a polycrisis — environmental, political, economic, cultural, institutional, and health — the old ways of relying solely on trade unions to influence workplace and state policies are not enough. New approaches are necessary to tackle those interconnected crises we face worldwide and within countries.

Class Awareness

A significant challenge in the working class's efforts to enhance their quality of life is that many workers are unaware that the underlying cause of their unfavourable working, living, and health conditions is the system they depend on — capitalism. Due to the lack of class consciousness, both as a class "in itself" and "for itself" (Marx 1847, 76–80), many workers fail to recognize capitalism as their main adversary. This absence of class awareness leads them admire capitalist ideas and practices. It is crucial to address this flaw in thinking and inspire workers and the masses to envision and strive for a healthier, more equitable world under a socialist system.

It is essential to understand that as economies evolved and more people joined the workforce, they encountered similar problems because of how capitalism worked. This situation united them against the wealthy capitalist class, even if they did not initially see it. However, through various struggles over time and space, they will realize they share common interests and come together with shared goals. This inevitable clash between classes is also a political fight (Marx 1847, 76–80). Understanding the battles between classes is critical for reaching socialism and health equity.

Trade Unions

Contemporary trade unions are fragmented and, therefore, weak. As such, they are easily overpowered by the combined forces of capital and the state. This power imbalance has made them retreat and assume a defeatist stance in economic and political struggles. Not surprisingly, they often rejoice over small wins through concessionary bargaining, thus applying the same subterfuge as the capitalists.

Specifically, trade unions' reluctance to use strike power to achieve bigger wins is partly due to many members struggling in the current environment. Strikes, once a powerful tool, now risk alienating the public, as seen in transport strikes. This situation creates a gap between workers' goals and public support. Strikes had some power when they stopped production, but when they stopped the buses from running, they alienated people. However, when an informed public backs strikes, they can be effective, benefiting both workers and communities, as seen in health workers' and nurses' strikes.

Unfortunately, today's trade unions increasingly concentrate power in top leaders' hands (Evans et al. 2023), moving away from participatory and democratic leadership. This hierarchical leadership worsens division among members and makes workers feel disenchanted with unions and politics. We must address this problem to bring back solidarity in unions and encourage people to be more involved in politics at all levels of society.

On the ground, frontline workers are unsure if their unions can improve their employment and living conditions, which is a big concern. For example, health care workers consider leaving work because they do not see improvements in concrete situations like low pay, excessive workload, and abuse (Wilson 2023). This reality underscores the need for honest, critical dialogue between union officials and the rank and file. Union leaders and organizers must initiate massive information, education, and workshop campaigns to reach and engage more members. Workers must become political activists.

In today's world, where awareness of social classes and the number of workers in trade unions are decreasing, it is vital to inspire, motivate, and empower people willing to challenge capitalism. We must educate, organize, and mobilize workers and the masses from all backgrounds politically. We must unite them under the flag of socialism — a movement driven by ordinary people and workers pushing for genuine democracy and fairness to improve life. This people's movement aims to make people and the planet healthier.

People Power

Throughout history, many people and communities have joined to change or replace capitalist systems with socialism. People's movements for emancipation from exploitation and oppression have been driven by workers, farmers, fishers, Indigenous Peoples, students, religious communities, and others who want to build socialism and be free. Recent people's power struggles have stood up to and defeated corporate and state forces (e.g., see Transnational Institute 2017, 2018). Ultimately, the determination of ordinary people decides what happens to their governments, countries, and the world.

People's movements worldwide show how the workers and the masses decisively act to change society and politics. In Canada, there have been movements such as the Winnipeg General Strike, Indigenous efforts to protect water and land, Idle No More, campaigns for disability rights and racial justice, climate activism, the Occupy Movement, Québec's Maple Spring, Ontario's Days of Action, the Alberta Nurses Strike, various health movements, and labour strikes. These efforts, aimed at improving working, living, and health conditions, provide valuable lessons for present and future struggles toward socialism and health equity.

Engaging Nurses in the Fight for Health Equity

As nurses — whether students, teachers, researchers, activists, practitioners, or policymakers — we should use the insights from this book to tackle health inequities. We must understand that health inequities stem from more than just individual lifestyle and behaviour; they are deeply influenced by societal systems that affect our lives and work as nurses. Effective nursing activism addresses issues like unhealthy workplaces, unstable housing, and unequal access to health services. Nursing is not just about caring for patients at the bedside; it requires understanding how economic, political, cultural, institutional, and environmental factors affect health. With this broader understanding, nurses can address the root causes of health inequities and push for an equitable health care system.

The nursing community, including unions and individual nurses, must actively engage in social activism and political actions to shape a fairer and better world. This commitment involves organizing rallies, participating in protests, and being ready to strike when necessary. Nurses exemplify empowered care through advocacy for meaningful health policy, giving a voice to marginalized communities, and challenging unjust societal norms (Falk-Rafael 2005, 220). This political stance is at the core of nursing, reflecting a dedication to social justice and health equity.

Nursing practice standards emphasize the need to address the root causes of health inequities. Thus, we must engage in political activism to advocate for economic and societal changes to improve health outcomes. Nursing activism means joining political campaigns with workers and community movements and confronting capitalism's ways. Despite the belief that nurses are not politically active, things are changing. Nurses and their unions are now more involved in political actions like protests and strikes. Globally, nurses are speaking out and acting against worsening working, living, and health conditions; they are increasingly standing up against exploitative and oppressive systems (Borras, Komakech, and Raphael 2023, 47). In Canada, five big unions — Ontario Council of Hospital Unions, Ontario Nurses Association, Ontario Public Service Employees Union, SEIU Healthcare, and Unifor — are actively fighting against health care privatization, staff shortages, and restrictive laws like Bill 124, showing growing dissatisfaction among workers.

Moreover, the Ontario Federation of Labour's Enough Is Enough campaign demands higher wages, affordable housing, stable rent prices, and increased taxes on large companies and banks (2023). In an initiative by the Ontario Health Coalition, 98% of people voted against for-profit health care (Shuttleworth 2023). These actions show that labour and health movements are committed to addressing the problems caused by capitalism, neocolonialism, racism, and sexism. Workers and the masses are determined to make big changes for better jobs, living conditions, and health.

Our Minimum Demands

There are many sound policy ideas to address health inequities, but big companies and politicians who support the current system are obstructing progress. Therefore, civil society groups, including workers and social movements, must continue to push leaders to make significant changes that address the root causes of health and health care inequities. This united effort needs to challenge the ways capitalism, neocolonialism, racism, and sexism create and maintain such inequities.

We must emphasize that the policy changes we are advocating for are based on socialist ideas and practices, not capitalist ones. The policy actions proposed below may seem like small changes within the prevailing governmental systems, but they are deeply rooted in socialist principles. This dual approach has a strategic goal: to make real and noticeable improvements within capitalism while setting the stage for socialism now and in the future. Socialist societies aim to meet people's needs, not make profits to satisfy private interests. Our demands that lean toward socialism should cover a wide range of areas, including but not limited to the following socialist policies:

Strengthen Working Conditions and Employment Standards

State policies should ensure that people have stable, full-time jobs with wages they can decently live on, fair treatment at work, equal pay for equal work, and transparent salary information. It is essential to have different kinds of leave available, such as sick leave for short-term illnesses, medical leave for serious health issues, family emergency leave, parental leave, compassionate care leave, and leave for bereavement. A robust employment insurance program is needed to deal with financial problems when workers lose jobs, become disabled, get older, or have health needs. Governments should make it easier for workers to join unions and protect their labour rights, including their right to strike. Following these policy suggestions is essential in tackling the main reasons behind health inequities related to employment. In Canada, the employment situation shows how urgent this is: more than 1.2 million are unemployed, and 3.7 million work part-time as of January 2024 (Statistics Canada 2024c, 11). Unstable jobs and not having a job result in lower incomes, more people living in poverty, and worsening health inequities.

Elevate Income and Social Support

Increasing income and social support is significant because having low income leads to poverty, which affects millions of people. Addressing this problem could make health better and fairer. For example, if health indicator rates for lower income people in Canada were the same as those for people with the highest incomes, about a million households would not have had food insecurity in 2011–12. In 2013, there could have been 673,700 fewer cases of diabetes (a 32.1% decrease), 580,700 fewer women with obesity (a 24.1% decrease), and 300 fewer babies dying (a 15.1% decrease) (CIHI 2015, 12–13). Higher incomes are crucial for better and fairer health because people can then afford quality food, housing, and health services. Moreover, when people are healthier, they can earn more money, which helps make the population healthier.

Advance Access to Socialized Housing

Improving public and social housing is vital because it directly impacts health. Unstable housing causes serious health problems, such as increased injuries, stress, and fatal heart issues (WHO 2018). In Canada, millions face housing insecurity, and 235,000 people experience homelessness every year (Gaetz, Dej, and Richter 2016, 12). If people in the four lowest income groups had housing security like those in the highest income group, there would have been 1.6 million fewer cases of housing insecurity in 2011 (CIHI 2015, 12). Thus, housing insecurity can be eradicated. Investing in social housing is not just about giving people a roof over their heads; it also improves their overall well-being by improving their living conditions. It is not just a matter of social policy but an intelligent move for public health.

Expand Access to Health Services

Expanding health care systems is critical to ensure that everyone gets the necessary care. In Canada, 3.4 million people over 12 say they did not get the health services they needed, significantly affecting people with lower incomes in 2014 (Statistics Canada 2016). In 2021, 85.5% reported having a regular health care provider, but 14.4%, or 4.7 million people, did not. Among those with a provider, 58.3% could secure an appointment within three days. However, nearly 2.5 million, or 7.9%, indicated unmet health care needs. These unmet needs were more prevalent in the Atlantic provinces compared to other regions (Statistics Canada 2024d, 39). In 2022, individuals with unmet health care needs increased to 9.2%, up from 7.9% in 2021 (Statistics Canada 2024e). If people from the four lowest income groups had the same access to care as people with the highest incomes, there would have been 14.6% fewer heart attack hospitalizations, 31.6% fewer hospital admissions because of alcohol, and 26.8% fewer hospital stays for mental health reasons in 2012 (CIHI 2015, 13).

We can close the gaps in health between different classes and groups by adding more services like pharmaceutical, dental, long-term, home, and mental health care. Ensuring everyone has health care access makes the population healthier, and healthy people take pressure off hospitals and other care facilities. Investing in health services is not just about health care — it is a wise move for making society healthier overall.

Beyond Policy Change Limitations

Adopting sound ideas from the Socialist Project Labour Movement Platform, we can focus on three urgent tasks to take meaningful actions within and beyond capitalism (the ideas in this section are from the Socialist Project 2023). These endeavours can lead us toward socialism and offer the best chance to reduce and eliminate health inequities: (1) cultivate class awareness and solidarity among diverse workers; (2) strengthen democratic representation and participation within labour movements; and (3) establish a genuine socialist political party.

Cultivate Class Awareness and Solidarity

Unions are essential for workers because they are the most organized group within the working classes. However, unions must change how they operate and use their power to maximize their potential. Currently, unions compete excessively, especially in recruiting new members, which weakens their collective power. Instead, they should support each other, particularly in bargaining with employers This solidaristic endeavour ensures workers understand their shared interests and goals of improving working, living, and health conditions.

Unions must change how they operate to make workers more aware of their shared aspirations and bond together. Specifically, unions should work together across sectors instead of focusing on one workplace at a time. For example, they can negotiate with large employers in the private service sector, strengthening their collective voice. When unions team up, they can make more extensive changes that benefit workers in different industries and even create positive impacts beyond workplaces, enhancing people's lives.

Furthermore, unions must support workers who are not part of a union. They can collaborate with organizations like the Workers' Action Centre in Toronto, the Montreal Immigrant Workers Centre, and the Workers' Organizing and Resource Centre in Winnipeg. Unions should leverage their power in negotiations to assist non-union workers in organizing. They should also encourage their members to engage in community issues such as housing, health care, education, and transportation — all connected to labour issues. Strikes should not just be about wages and benefits; they should also be used to protect workers' rights and defend and expand laws like the National Housing Strategy Act and the Canada Health Act.

Unions must also stand up for immigrant workers regardless of their legal status. Many immigrants come to Canada from the Global South to escape harsh economic conditions created by global capitalism but face even more unfair treatment in workplaces in the Global North. They must adopt a broader approach, supporting Indigenous rights and land struggles and combating racism, sexism, ableism, ageism, colonialism, and imperialism. Unions must also work for environmental and health justice.

Importantly, unions must engage in political action to fight oppression and push for social justice. They should closely collaborate with other social movements that strive for social justice. Recognizing the interconnectedness of workers' struggles, unions should also support labour movements in other countries. Victories for workers elsewhere can inspire workers anywhere. Unions should advocate for the right of each nation to self-determination and promote international solidarity, as unity among workers transcends national borders. International worker unity is essential since global capitalism influences and shapes social and health inequities within a country.

Strengthen Democratic Representation and Participation

Making labour movements more democratic involves creating safe spaces where everyone feels encouraged to express their views instead of a few people making all the decisions. During tough times, union leaders often make decisions without broad involvement, assuming they know what is best for the organization. For leaders to truly represent their members, they must listen to feedback, which empowers members and strengthens the union by considering diverse views.

Union elections are infrequent, and challenging current leaders is seen as disloyalty rather than a way to ensure accountability. Presently, union participation usually means agreeing with top leaders, which is unhelpful. Real union democracy goes beyond voting or following a leader's vision. Thus, members must be encouraged to get involved and speak up about what matters to them, not just follow the leaders. Leaders do not own their organizations nor possess all the knowledge and skills to address labour and health issues. In fact, some members are more visionary than their leaders. Unions exist because of their members; leaders should remember this and be willing to step down when necessary. Sometimes, leaders stay in power too long, focusing more on retaining their position than benefiting the union. They also resist new ideas and adhere to outdated theories and practices, blocking essential changes that could help the labour movement grow.

Real democracy in unions is built when workers unite and fight for their rights. Without constantly improving democratic practices in the labour movement, unions risk losing members' passion, commitment, and creativity. They must give union members more opportunities to develop their capacities and leadership skills and involve them in all union activities. This way, they can generate new ideas to challenge the status quo. Unions should create more opportunities for members to connect, share ideas, discuss issues, and collaborate with non-union workers and community groups focused on workers' concerns.

Importantly, unions must actively combat discrimination within unions and workers' movements, ensuring everyone, regardless of race, gender, disability, or age, can fully participate and become leaders in the union and community. They must scrutinize union structures to ensure members have more influence in choosing their leaders. Top-down leadership is not only undemocratic but also authoritarian.

Establish a Genuine Socialist Political Party

Workers need more than just unions to form a solid political group that can challenge capitalist systems. While unions bring workers together, their ability to unite different groups against capitalism is limited. Unions can help workers understand their shared interests, strengthen their unity, and improve democracy, but a political party specifically for workers is crucial. Achieving socialism and health equity requires a socialist political party.

A socialist political party supports workers and other social movements through ongoing discussions and innovative approaches to learning, development, and improvement. This continuous reciprocal process strengthens us as we work toward a society based on socialist ideas and practices. To build a robust socialist party, workers and civil society groups must continuously collaborate, engage in critical dialogue, and unite against capitalism while advocating for socialism.

Conclusions

Health inequities are serious problems caused by a few entities controlling people's ways of thinking and doing things. Despite the existence of research-backed ideas to prevent such inequities, these problems persist due to exploitative/oppressive social systems. This book shows that addressing the economic, political, cultural, institutional, and environmental dimensions of life is a sensible way to get rid of health inequities.

This book reveals the root causes of health inequities: unequal wealth and power among policy advocates, big businesses dominating health politics, and neoliberal state policies. It demonstrates how the power, interests, and ideology of capital override socialist policies like fair wealth distribution, socialized housing, universal health care, and improved work conditions. Additionally, the book highlights that the capitalist system, integrally connected with historical colonialism, racism, and sexism, forms barriers to addressing health inequities. It adds depth to discussions on inequities related to class, race, and gender, offering both theoretical and practical approaches to health inequities. This book stimulates critical dialogue toward socialism and health equity. This book unveils the following:

1. Contrary to its stellar international reputation, entrenched inequities plague Canada's health care system.
2. Capitalism fundamentally drives health inequities.
3. The interconnection of capitalism with colonialism, imperialism, racism, and sexism exacerbates health inequities.
4. State policies that undermine public services worsen health inequities.
5. Imbalances in wealth and power among capital, state, and civil society skew health policy outcomes in favour of capital.
6. Capitalist agendas dominate policymaking, obstructing policies that would otherwise enhance the quality of life for workers and communities.

7. Ruling governments enact neoliberal policies, solidifying a mutualistic symbiotic relationship between the state and capital, consolidating wealth and power among the elite, and resulting in inequitable distribution of the social determinants of health.
8. Corporate and neoliberal actors' immense power and influence prevent evidence-based policies that could substantially address social and health inequities.
9. Capital interests prioritize profit over policies that could enhance ecological, societal, and human well-being.
10. The capitalist class's ideology eclipses research and policy initiatives capable of preventing and reducing health inequities.
11. Weaknesses within trade unions and divisions among social movements contribute to the unequal distribution of health-related social factors.
12. Socialism is the alternative road toward social justice and health equity.

Addressing health inequities requires a solid coalition of anti-capitalist and socialist individuals and groups committed to advocating for fair and equitable public policies. These socialist-oriented policies must redistribute wealth and power from Big Capital to workers and the masses, bridging gender and racial inequality. Key to preventing health inequities is a combination of information, education, advocacy, organization, and mobilization for systemic change that will free workers, women, racialized groups, and other exploited/oppressed populations from the grips of the capital-state alliance. Realizing health equity means fighting against capitalism — within and outside the state — to establish socialism.

Socialism demands a radical restructuring of production and industry management, shifting control from individual competitors to a collective society operating for the common good. With everyone's involvement, socialism entails planned production for public benefit, replacing competition with collaboration. In this new societal order, communal ownership of goods and services replaces private property. This dissolution of private property epitomizes the societal revolution driven by industrial progress (Marx and Engels [1848] 1964). Embraced by proletarian socialists, this seismic shift aims to structure society for communal benefit over individual gain.

Workers and masses, arise!
Exploited and oppressed people around the world, unite!
We have a world to win!

References

Acheson, David. 1998. *Independent Inquiry into Inequalities in Health: Report*. HM Stationery Office.
Aggleton, Peter. 1990. *Health (Society Now)*. Routledge.
Anderson, Ian, Sue Crengle, Martina Leialoha Kamaka, et al. 2006. "Indigenous Health in Australia, New Zealand, and the Pacific." *The Lancet* 367, 9524. https://doi.org/10.1016/S0140-6736(06)68773-4.
Anderson, Sarah. 2023. *Executive Excess 2023*. Institute for Policy Studies. https://ips-dc.org/wp-content/uploads/2023/08/EE23-FINAL-aug-23-23.pdf.
Armitage, Karen J., Lawrence J. Schneiderman, and Robert A. Bass. 1979. "Response of Physicians to Medical Complaints in Men and Women." *JAMA* 241, 20. https://doi.org/10.1001/jama.1979.03290460050020.
Armstrong, Pat, and Hugh Armstrong. 2003. *Wasting Away: The Undermining of Canadian Health Care*. Oxford University Press.
Bailey, Zinzi D., Nancy Krieger, Madina Agénor, et al. 2017. "Structural Racism and Health Inequities in the USA: Evidence and Interventions." *The Lancet* 389, 10077. https://doi.org/10.1016/S0140-6736(17)30569-X.
Bambra, Clare, Debbie Fox, and Alex Scott-Samuel. 2005. "Towards a Politics of Health." *Health Promotion International* 20, 2. https://doi.org/10.1093/heapro/dah608.
Banting, Keith, and John Myles (eds.). 2013. *Inequality and the Fading of Redistributive Politics*. UBC Press.
Baum, Fran. 2007. "Cracking the Nut of Health Equity: Top Down and Bottom Up Pressure for Action on the Social Determinants of Health." *Promotion and Education* 14, 2. https://doi.org/10.1177/10253823070140022002.
Baum, Frances E., Paul Laris, Matthew Fisher, et al. 2013. "Never Mind the Logic, Give Me the Numbers: Former Australian Health Ministers' Perspectives on the Social Determinants of Health." *Social Science and Medicine* 87. https://doi.org/10.1016/j.socscimed.2013.03.033.
Baum, Fran, Belinda Townsend, Matthew Fisher, et al. 2020. "Creating Political Will for Action on Health Equity: Practical Lessons for Public Health Policy Actors." *International Journal of Health Policy and Management* 11, 7. https://doi.org/10.34172/IJHPM.2020.233.
Beattie, Samantha, and Bobby Hristova. 2023. "Ontario NDP Kicks Hamilton MPP Sarah Jama from Caucus after Controversial Gaza Comments." *CBC News*, October 23, 2023. https://www.cbc.ca/news/canada/hamilton/jama-ndp-caucus-1.7005056.

Béland, Daniel, and Robert H. Cox. 2016. "Ideas as Coalition Magnets: Coalition Building, Policy Entrepreneurs, and Power Relations." *Journal of European Public Policy* 23, 3.

Benach, Joan, Alejandra Vives, Gemma Tarafa, et al. 2016. "What Should We Know about Precarious Employment and Health in 2025? Framing the Agenda for the Next Decade of Research." *International Journal of Epidemiology* 45, 1. https://doi.org/10.1093/ije/dyv342.

Berman, Gabrielle, and Yin Paradies. 2010. "Racism, Disadvantage and Multiculturalism: Towards Effective Anti-Racist Praxis." *Ethnic and Racial Studies* 33, 2.

Black, Douglas, J.N. Morris, Cyril Smith, et al. 1992. "The Black Report." In *Inequalities in Health: The Black Report and the Health Divide*, edited by Peter Townsend, Nick Davidson, and Margaret Whitehead. Penguin.

Block, Sheila, Grace-Edward Galabuzi, and Ricardo Tranjan. 2019. *Canada's Colour Coded Income Inequality*. Canadian Centre for Policy Alternatives. https://policyalternatives.ca/sites/default/files/uploads/publications/National%20Office/2019/12/Canada%27s%20Colour%20Coded%20Income%2Inequality.pdf.

Blyth, Mark M. 1997. "'Any More Bright Ideas?' The Ideational Turn of Comparative Political Economy." *Comparative Politics* 29.

Boniol, Mathieu, Michelle McIsaac, Lihui Xu, et al. 2019. *Gender Equity in the Health Workforce: Analysis of 104 Countries*. World Health Organization. https://iris.who.int/bitstream/handle/10665/311314/WHO-HIS-HWF-Gender-WP1-2019.1-eng.pdf?sequence=1.

Borras, Arnel M. 2016. "Towards Equitable Health Policy: A Critical Approach to Canadian Housing Insecurity and Homelessness as Informed by Political Economy and Social Determinants of Health." Master's Major Research Paper, York University. YorkSpace. https://yorkspace.library.yorku.ca/server/api/core/bitstreams/od9d5669-0b40-4552-9fc1-a21ab56a26f1/content.

———. 2021. "Toward an Intersectional Approach to Health Justice." *International Journal of Health Services* 51, 2. https://doi.org/10.1177/0020731420981857.

———. 2022. "Tackling Health Inequalities through Public Policy Action: Insights from Canadian Policy Academics, Activists, and Advocates." Doctoral dissertation, School of Health Policy and Management, York University, Toronto. https://yorkspace.library.yorku.ca/items/da139d31-0f00-4411-a797-af45e397260b.

———. 2023. "The Challenge of Exposing and Ending Health Inequalities Through Social and Policy Change: Canadian Experiences." *International Journal of Social Determinants of Health and Health Services* 53, 2. https://doi.org/10.1177/27551938221148376.

Borras, Arnel M., Morris Komakech, and Dennis Raphael. 2023. "Policy-Related Homelessness Discourses in Canada: Implications for Nursing Research, Practice, and Advocacy." *Witness: The Canadian Journal of Critical Nursing Discourse* 5, 1. https://doi.org/10.25071/2291-5796.145.

Borras, Jana, Luin Goldring, and Patricia Landolt. 2021. *Pandemic Precarities: Immigration Status, Work, Housing, and Health among Current and Former*

Non-Status Residents of Toronto. FGJ Refugee Centre and CEP Project. https://hdl.handle.net/1807/110639.

Bryant, Toba. 2016. *Health Policy in Canada*, 2nd ed. Canadian Scholars' Press Inc.

Bryant, Toba, and Dennis Raphael. 2016. "Opening Policy Windows with Evidence and Citizen Engagement: Addressing the Social Determinants of Health Inequalities." In *Creating and Implementing Public Policy: Cross-Sectoral Debates*, edited by Gemma Carey, Kathy Landvogt, and Jo Barraket, 25–40. Routledge.

———. 2020. *The Politics of Health in the Canadian Welfare State*. Canadian Scholars' Press.

Bushnik, Tracey, Michael Tjepkema, and Laurent Martel. 2020. "Socioeconomic Disparities in Life and Health Expectancy among the Household Population in Canada." *Health Reports* 31. https://www.doi.org/10.25318/82-003-x202000100001-eng.

Cairney, Paul, and Christopher M. Weible. 2015. "Comparing and Contrasting Peter Hall's Paradigms and Ideas with the Advocacy Coalition Framework." In *Policy Paradigms in Theory and Practice*, edited by John Hogan and Michael Howlett, 83–99. Palgrave.

Canadian Dental Association. 2023. "The Canadian Dental Association Welcomes Significant Funding for Dental Care." March 28. https://www.cda-adc.ca/EN/about/media_room/news_releases/2023/03_28_CDA_welcomes_significant_funding_dental_care.asp#:~:text=The%20Canadian%20Dental%20Association%20(CDA,Dental%20Care%20Plan%20(CDCP).

Carey, Gemma, and Brad Crammond. 2015. "Action on the Social Determinants of Health: Views from Inside the Policy Process." *Social Science and Medicine* 128. https://doi.org/10.1016/j.socscimed.2015.01.024.

Carroll, William K., and J.P. Sapinski. 2018. *Organizing the 1%: How Corporate Power Works*. Fernwood Publishing.

Cawson, Alan. 1978. "Pluralism, Corporatism and the Role of the State." *Government and Opposition* 13, 2. https://doi.org/10.1111/j.1477-7053.1978.tb00542.x.

Centers for Disease Control and Prevention. n.d. "COVID-19 Hospitalization and Death by Race/Ethnicity." https://stacks.cdc.gov/view/cdc/91857.

Chadwick, Edwin. 1842. *Report on the Sanitary Condition of the Labouring Population and on the Means of Its Improvement*. https://s3.amazonaws.com/aspphwebassets/delta-omega/archives/ChadwickClassic.pdf.

Chaufan, Claudia, Meagan Davis, and Sophia Constantino. 2011. "The Twin Epidemics of Poverty and Diabetes: Understanding Diabetes Disparities in a Low-Income Latino and Immigrant Neighborhood." *Journal of Community Health* 36. https://link.springer.com/article/10.1007/s10900-011-9406-2.

CHC (Canadian Health Coalition). 2016. "History of Canada's Public Health Care." https://archive.healthcoalition.ca/tools-and-resources/history-of-canadas-public-health-care/.

Cheff, Rebecca. 2017. *Making Room for Health Equity*. Wellesley Institute. https://www.wellesleyinstitute.com/wp-content/uploads/2017/06/Making-Room-for-Health-Equity-Final.pdf.

Chung, Hannah, Kinwah Fung, Laura E. Ferreira-Legere, et al. 2020. *COVID-19 Laboratory Testing in Ontario: Patterns of Testing and Characteristics of Individuals*

Tested, as of April 30, 2020. ON: ICES. https://www.ices.on.ca/publications/research-reports/covid-19-laboratory-testing-in-ontario-patterns-of-testing-and-characteristics-of-individuals-tested-as-of-april-30-2020/.

CIHI (Canadian Institute for Health Information). 2015. *Trends in Income-Related Health Inequalities in Canada*. https://www.cihi.ca/sites/default/files/document/summary_report_inequalities_2015_en.pdf.

———. 2019. *Health System Resources for Mental Health and Addictions Care in Canada*. https://www.cihi.ca/sites/default/files/document/mental-health-chartbook-report-2019-en-web.pdf.

———. 2020a. *Pandemic Experience in the Long-term Care: How Does Canada Compare with Other Countries?* https://www.cihi.ca/sites/default/files/document/COVID-19-rapid-response-long-term-care-snapshot-en.pdf.

———. 2020b. "1 in 3 Unpaid Caregivers in Canada Are Distressed." https://www.cihi.ca/en/1-in-3-unpaid-caregivers-in-canada-are-distressed.

———. 2021. "Long-Term Care Homes in Canada: How Many and Who Owns Them?" https://www.cihi.ca/en/long-term-care-homes-in-canada-how-many-and-who-owns-them.

———. 2022a. "A Lens on the Supply of Canada's Health Workforce." https://www.cihi.ca/en/health-workforce-in-canada-in-focus-including-nurses-and-physicians/a-lens-on-the-supply-of-canadas.

———. 2022b. "Health Care Provider Experiences During the COVID-19 Pandemic." https://www.cihi.ca/en/health-workforce-in-canada-in-focus-including-nurses-and-physicians/health-care-provider.

———. 2022c. "Health Workforce in Canada: In Focus (Including Nurses and Physicians)." https://www.cihi.ca/en/health-workforce-in-canada-in-focus-including-nurses-and-physicians.

———. 2023a. "National Health Expenditure Trends, 2023 — Snapshot." Accessed May 31, 2024. https://www.cihi.ca/en/national-health-expenditure-trends-2023-snapshot.

———. 2023b. "Who Is Paying for These Services? https://www.cihi.ca/en/who-is-paying-for-these-services.

———. 2024. "Supply and Distribution." https://www.cihi.ca/en/the-state-of-the-health-workforce-in-canada-2022/supply-and-distribution.

City of Toronto. 2023. "Toronto Public Health Releases 2022 Data for Deaths of People Experiencing Homelessness." *Toronto Public Health*, March 17.

———. n.d. "COVID-19 Infection in Toronto: Ethno-Racial Identity and Income." https://www.toronto.ca/community-people/health-wellness-care/health-programs-advice/respiratory-viruses/COVID-19/COVID-19-pandemic-data/COVID-19-archived-dashboards/COVID-19-ethno-racial-identity-income/.

Clark, Anna. 2011. "Domestic Violence, Past and Present." *Journal of Women's History* 23, 3. https://doi.org/10.1353/jowh.2011.0032.

Clarke, John. 2021. "Social Democracy Doesn't Deliver." *Counterfire*. December 18. https://www.counterfire.org/article/social-democracy-doesn-t-deliver/.

CMHC (Canada Mortgage and Housing Corporation). 2011. *Canadian Housing Observer 2011*. https://publications.gc.ca/collections/collection_2012/schl-cmhc/N-1-2011-eng.pdf.

____. 2018. *Housing Observer 2018 – Digest 2016 and 2017.* https://eppdscrmssa01.blob.core.windows.net/cmhcprodcontainer/sf/project/archive/publications/canadian_housing_observer/observer-compilation-2017-en.pdf.

____. 2020a. *Characteristics of Households in Core Housing Need: Canada, P/T, CMAS; Characteristics of Households in Core Housing Need Canada, 2001.* https://www.cmhc-schl.gc.ca/professionals/housing-markets-data-and-research/housing-data/data-tables/household-characteristics/characteristics-households-core-housing-need-canada-pt-cmas.

____. 2020b. *Characteristics of Households in Core Housing Need: Canada, Provinces/Territories, Census Metropolitan Areas; Characteristics of Households in Core Housing Need Canada, 2016.* Accessed August 30, 2023. https://www.cmhc-schl.gc.ca/professionals/housing-markets-data-and-research/housing-data/data-tables/household-characteristics/characteristics-households-core-housing-need-canada-pt-cmas.

____. 2022. *Adequacy, Suitability and Affordability Statistics for Visible Minority Groups.* Accessed March 20, 2024. https://www.cmhc-schl.gc.ca/professionals/housing-markets-data-and-research/housing-data/data-tables/household-characteristics/appendix-3-adequacy-suitability-affordability-visible-minority.

Coffey, Clare, Patricia Espinoza Revollo, Rowan Harvey, et al. 2020. *Time to Care: Unpaid and Underpaid Care Work and the Global Inequality Crisis.* Oxfam. https://oxfamilibrary.openrepository.com/bitstream/handle/10546/620928/bp-time-to-care-inequality-200120-en.pdf.

Cohen, Benita E., and Shelley G. Marshall. 2017. "Does Public Health Advocacy Seek to Redress Health Inequities? A Scoping Review." *Health and Social Care in the Community* 25, 2. https://doi.org/10.1111/hsc.12320.

Cortes, Kassandra, and Leah Smith. 2022. "Pharmaceutical Access and Use during the Pandemic." Statistics Canada. https://www150.statcan.gc.ca/n1/pub/75-006-x/2022001/article/00011-eng.htm.

COVID Tracking Project. n.d. "The COVID Racial Data Tracker." https://covidtracking.com/race.

Dahl, Robert A. 1961. *Who Governs? Power and Democracy in an American City.* Yale University Press.

____. 1984. "Polyarchy, Pluralism, and Scale." *Scandinavian Political Studies* 7, 4. https://doi.org/10.1111/j.1467-9477.1984.tb00304.x.

Davis, Mike. 2017. *Planet of Slums.* Verso.

De Stefano, Valerio. 2016. "The Rise of the 'Just-in-Time Workforce': On-Demand Work, Crowdwork, and Labor Protection in the Gig-Economy." *Comparative Labor Law and Policy Journal* 37, 3.

Doucet, Brandon. 2023. *About Canada: Dental Care*, Vol. 14. Fernwood Publishing.

Doyal, Lesley. 1995. *What Makes Women Sick: Gender and the Political Economy of Health.* Bloomsbury Publishing.

Dryden, Joel, and Sarah Rieger. 2020. "Inside the Slaughterhouse." *CBC News*, May 6. https://newsinteractives.cbc.ca/longform/cargill-covid19-outbreak.

Dungca, Nancy, and Colin Healey. 2023. "Revealing The Smithsonian's 'Racial Brain Collection.'" *Washington Post*, August 14.

Duong, Diana. 2023. "Feds Propose $196B Health Funding Deal with Few Strings Attached." *CMAJ* 195, 8: E311-E312. https://doi.org/10.1503/cmaj.1096040.
Dye, Thomas. 2017. *Understanding Public Policy*, 15th ed. Pearson Education, Inc.
Edwards, Michael. 2019. *Housing Conditions of Visible Minority Households*. CMHC. https://publications.gc.ca/collections/collection_2019/schl-cmhc/nh70-1/NH70-1-6-2019-eng.pdf.
Ehrenreich, Barbara, and Deirdre English. 1973. *Witches, Midwives, and Nurses: A History of Women Healers*. Lunaria Press.
Engels, Friedrich. 1845. *The Condition of the Working Class in England*. Accessed November 8, 2023. https://www.marxists.org/archive/marx/works/download/pdf/condition-working-class-england.pdf.
Esping-Andersen, Gøsta. 1990. *The Three Worlds of Welfare Capitalism*. Polity Press.
Evans, Bryan, Carlo Fanelli, Leo Panitch, et al. 2023. "To Renew Working Class Resistance, the Labour Movement Must Be Democratized." *Canadian Dimension*. https://canadiandimension.com/articles/view/to-renew-working-class-resistance-the-labour-movement-must-be-democratized.
Exworthy, Mark. 2002. "The 'Second Black Report'? The Acheson Report as Another Opportunity to Tackle Health Inequalities." *Contemporary British History* 16, 3. https://doi.org/10.1080/713999459.
Exworthy, Mark, Lee Berney, and Martin Powell. 2002. "How Great Expectations in Westminster May Be Dashed Locally: The Local Implementation of National Policy on Health Inequalities." *Policy and Politics* 30, 1. https://doi.org/10.1332/0305573022501584.
Exworthy, Mark, David Blane, and Michael Marmot. 2003. "Tackling Health Inequalities in the United Kingdom: The Progress and Pitfalls of Policy." *Health Services Research* 38, 6p2. https://doi.org/10.1111/j.1475-6773.2003.00208.x.
Falk-Rafael, Adeline. 2005. "Speaking Truth to Power: Nursing's Legacy and Moral Imperative." *Advances in Nursing Science* 28, 3. https://doi.org/10.1097/00012272-200507000-00004.
Fanon, Frantz. 1963. *The Wretched of the Earth*. Grove Press.
FAO, IFAD, UNICEF, WFP, and WHO. 2023. "The State of Food Security and Nutrition in the World 2023. Urbanization, Agrifood Systems Transformation and Healthy Diets across the Rural–Urban Continuum." Rome: FAO. https://doi.org/10.4060/cc3017en.
FAO (Financial Accountability Office of Ontario). 2023. "Ontario Health Sector: Spending Plan Review." https://www.fao-on.org/en/Blog/Publications/health-2023.
Fincher, Contessa, Joyce E. Williams, Vicky MacLean, et al. 2004. "Racial Disparities in Coronary Heart Disease: A Sociological View of the Medical Literature on Physician Bias." *Ethnicity and Disease* 14, 3. https://www.jstor.org/stable/48666472.
Finkel, Alvin. 2018. *Compassion: A Global History of Social Policy*. Red Globe Press.
Flood, Colleen M., Sara Allin, Sarah L. Lazin, et al. 2023. "Toward a Universal Dental Care Plan: Policy Options for Canada." *IRPP Insight* 46. https://irpp.org/wp-content/uploads/2023/06/Toward-a-Universal-Dental-Care-Plan-Policy-Options-for-Canada.pdf.

Fox, Jonathan. 1993. *The Politics of Food in Mexico: State Power and Social Mobilization*. Cornell University Press. https://jonathan-fox.org/wp-content/uploads/2018/12/Fox_The_Politics_of_Food_in_Mexico.pdf.

Fraser, Nancy. 2023. *Cannibal Capitalism: How Our System Is Devouring Democracy, Care, and the Planet — and What We Can Do About It*. Verso Books.

Fry, Sarah, Bill Cousins, and Ken Olivola. 2002. *Health of Children Living in Urban Slums in Asia and the Near East: Review of Existing Literature and Data*. Environmental Health Project, US Agency for International Development. https://pdf.usaid.gov/pdf_docs/pnacq101.pdf

Gaetz, Stephen, Erin Dej, and Tim Richter. 2016. *The State of Homelessness in Canada 2016*. Canadian Observatory on Homelessness Press. https://yorkspace.library.yorku.ca/server/api/core/bitstreams/5b919175-e7fc-4a20-8553-2a8c774a37be/content.

Gielen, Andrea C., Patricia J. O'Campo, Ruth R. Faden, et al. 1994. "Interpersonal Conflict and Physical Violence during the Childbearing Year." *Social Science and Medicine* 39, 6. https://doi.org/10.1016/0277-9536(94)90039-6.

Gilroy, Paul. 2021. "Introduction: Race Is the Prism." In *Selected Writings on Race and Difference: Stuart Hall*, 1–19. Duke University Press.

Gindin, Sam. 2023. "The Power of Deep Organizing." *The Bullet*. https://socialistproject.ca/2017/01/b1353/.

Goering, Paula, Scott Veldhuizen, Aimee Watson, et al. 2014. *National At Home/Chez Soi Final Report*. Mental Health Commission of Canada. https://mentalhealthcommission.ca/wp-content/uploads/2021/09/mhcc_at_home_report_national_cross-site_eng_2_0.pdf.

Government of Canada. 2018a. *Key Health Inequalities in Canada: A National Portrait*. Public Health Agency of Canada. https://www.canada.ca/content/dam/phac-aspc/documents/services/publications/science-research/key-health-inequalities-canada-national-portrait-executive-summary/key_health_inequalities_full_report-eng.pdf.

———. 2018b. *Canada's National Housing Strategy: A Place to Call Home*. https://publications.gc.ca/collections/collection_2018/edsc-esdc/Em12-54-2018-eng.pdf.

———. 2019. "Canada's Health Care System: Evolution of Our Health Care System." https://www.canada.ca/en/health-canada/services/health-care-system/reports-publications/health-care-system/canada.html.

———. 2023. "Prescription Drug Pricing and Costs." https://www.canada.ca/en/health-canada/services/health-care-system/pharmaceuticals/costs-prices.html.

GOV.UK. 2023. "NHS Workforce: 8: By Ethnicity and Grade." https://www.ethnicity-facts-figures.service.gov.uk/workforce-and-business/workforce-diversity/nhs-workforce/latest/#by-ethnicity-and-grade-managers-and-senior-managers.

Gramsci, Antonio. 1971. *Selections from the Prison Notebooks of Antonio Gramsci*. Edited and translated by Quentin Hoare and Geoffrey Nowell Smith. https://ia600506.us.archive.org/19/items/AntonioGramsciSelectionsFromThePrisonNotebooks/Antonio-Gramsci-Selections-from-the-Prison-Notebooks.pdf

Gundersen, Craig, Valerie Tarasuk, Joyce Cheng, et al. 2018. "Food Insecurity Status and Mortality among Adults in Ontario, Canada." *PLoS ONE* 13, 8: e0202642. https://doi.org/10.1371/journal.pone.0202642.

Hahmann, Tara, and Huda Masoud. 2023. *Housing Experiences and Measures of Health and Well-being Among First Nations People Living Off Reserve, Métis and Inuit: Findings from the 2018 Canadian Housing Survey*. Statistics Canada. April 4.

Hall, Peter A. 1993. "Policy Paradigms, Social Learning, and the State: The Case of Economic Policymaking in Britain." *Comparative Politics*. https://doi.org/10.2307/422246.

Hall, Peter A., and Michèle Lamont (eds.). 2013. *Social Resilience in the Neoliberal Era*. Cambridge University Press.

Hall, Stuart. 1997/2021. "Race, the Floating Signifier: What More Is There to Say About 'Race'?" In *Selected Writings on Race and Difference*, 350–373. Duke University Press.

Harvey, David. 2005. *The New Imperialism*. Oxford University Press.

———. 2007. *A Brief History of Neoliberalism*. Oxford University Press.

Heikkila, Tanya, and Paul Cairney. 2014. "A Comparison of Theories of the Policy Process." In *Theories of the Policy Process*, edited by Paul A. Sabatier and Christopher M. Weible, 301–327. Routledge. https://doi.org/10.4324/9780429494284-9.

Herr, Harvey, and Guenter Karl. 2002. "Estimating Global Slum Dwellers: Monitoring the Millennium Development Goal 7, Target 11." Monitoring Systems Branch, Global Urban Observatory, UN-HABITAT, Nairobi.

Heywood, Andrew. 2017. *Political Ideologies: An Introduction*. Macmillan International Higher Education.

Homeless Hub. n.d. "Canada Mortgage and Housing Corporation: Investment in Affordable Housing (2011–2014)." https://www.homelesshub.ca/resource/investment-affordable-housing-2011-2014.

Hulchanski, J. David, Philippa Campsie, Shirley B.Y. Chau, et al. 2009. *Finding Home: Policy Options for Addressing Homelessness in Canada*. Canadian Observatory on Homelessness.

International Labour Office. 2020. *ILO Monitor: COVID-19 and the World of Work. Fifth Edition. Estimates and Analysis*. https://www.oitcinterfor.org/sites/default/files/file_publicacion/5th_monitor.pdf.

John, Jipson, and Jitheesh P.M. 2019. "'The Neoliberal Project Is Alive But Has Lost Its Legitimacy': David Harvey." *The Wire*, February 9. https://thewire.in/economy/david-harvey-marxist-scholar-neo-liberalism.

Jones, Charles. 1984. *An Introduction to the Study of Public Policy*, 3rd ed. Brooks/Cole Publishing Company.

Kelley, Jacob, and Andrea H. Arce-Trigatti. 2021. "Heteropatriarchy." In *Encyclopedia of Queer Studies in Education*, edited by Kamden K. Strunk and Stephanie A. Shelton, 256–259. Leiden, Netherlands: Brill.

King, Robin L. 2016. "The Hidden Pockets in Toronto Where Gentrification Is Really Happening." *Toronto Star*, September 13.

Kingdon, John W. 1984/2014. *Agendas, Alternatives, and Public Policies*, 2nd ed. Pearson.

Kirby, James B., Gregg Taliaferro, and Samuel H. Zuvekas. 2006. "Explaining Racial and Ethnic Disparities in Health Care." *Medical Care* 44, 5. http://www.jstor.org/stable/3768359.

Labonté, Ronald, and David Stuckler. 2015. "The Rise of Neoliberalism: How Bad Economics Imperils Health and What to Do about It." *Journal of Epidemiology and Community Health* 70, 3. https://doi.org/10.1136/jech-2015-206295.

Langille, David. 2016. "Follow the Money: How Business and Politics Define Our Health." In *Social Determinants of Health: Canadian Perspectives*, edited by Dennis Raphael, 470–490. Canadian Scholars' Press.

Lasswell, Harold D. 1958. *Politics: Who Gets What, When, How*. The World Publishing Company.

Laurie, Melissa, and Rosalind P. Petchesky. 2008. "Gender, Health, and Human Rights in Sites of Political Exclusion." *Global Public Health* 3, S1. https://doi.org/10.1080/17441690801892125.

Lebowitz, Michael. 2023. "What Every Child Should Know About Marx's Theory of Value." *Monthly Review*.

Legislative Assembly of Ontario. 2023. "Bill 60, Your Health Act, 2023." https://www.ola.org/en/legislative-business/bills/parliament-43/session-1/bill-60.

Lindblom, Charles E. 1959. "The Science of 'Muddling Through.'" *Public Administration Review* 19, 2. https://www.jstor.org/stable/973677.

———. 1982. "The Market as Prison." *The Journal of Politics* 44, 2. https://doi.org/10.2307/2130588.

Logan, Trevon. 2024. "American Slavery Wasn't Just a White Man's Business – New Research Shows How White Women Profited, Too." *The Conversation*, June 10.

Lorde, Audre. 2018. *The Master's Tools Will Never Dismantle the Master's House*. Penguin.

Macdonald, David. 2018. *Born to Win*. Canadian Centre for Policy Alternatives. https://policyalternatives.ca/sites/default/files/uploads/publications/National%20Office/2018/07/Born%20to%20Win.pdf.

———. 2024. *How the Public Sector Is Fighting Income Inequality (And Why It's Still Not Enough)*. Canadian Centre for Policy Alternatives. https://policyalternatives.ca/sites/default/files/uploads/publications/National%20Office/2024/02/how-public-sector-is-fighting-income-inequality.pdf.

Mackenbach, Johan P. 2011. "Can We Reduce Health Inequalities? An Analysis of the English Strategy (1997–2010)." *Journal of Epidemiology and Community Health* 65, 7. https://doi.org/10.1136/jech.2010.128280.

Macnaughton, Eric, Geoffrey Nelson, and Paula Goering. 2013. "Bringing Politics and Evidence Together: Policy Entrepreneurship and the Conception of the At Home/Chez Soi Housing First Initiative for Addressing Homelessness and Mental Illness in Canada." *Social Science and Medicine* 82. https://doi.org/10.1016/j.socscimed.2013.01.033.

Macrotrends. n.d.a. "Canada Infant Mortality Rate 1950–2024." https://www.macrotrends.net/global-metrics/countries/CAN/canada/infant-mortality-rate.

———. n.d.b. "Canada Life Expectancy 1950–2024." https://www.macrotrends.net/global-metrics/countries/CAN/canada/life-expectancy#:~:text=The%20current%20life%20expectancy%20for,a%200.18%25%20increase%20from%202021.

Marchildon, Gregory P., Sara Allin, and Sherry Merkur. 2020. "Canada: Health System Review." *Health Systems in Transition* 22, 3. https://iris.who.int/bitstream/handle/10665/336311/HiT-22-3-2020-eng.pdf.
Marx, Karl. 1847. *The Poverty of Philosophy: Answer to the Philosophy of Poverty by M. Proudhon.* Progress Publishers. https://www.marxists.org/archive/marx/works/download/pdf/Poverty-Philosophy.pdf.
____. 1867. *Capital: A Critique of Political Economy. Das Kapital.* Progress Publishers.
Marx, Karl, and Friedrich Engels. [1848] 1964. *The Communist Manifesto.* Simon and Schuster, Inc.
Mazurek, Jacek M., John Wood, Donald J. Blackley, et al. 2018. "Coal Workers' Pneumoconiosis–Attributable Years of Potential Life Lost to Life Expectancy and Potential Life Lost before Age 65 Years — United States, 1999–2016." *Morbidity and Mortality Weekly Report* 67, 30. https://www.cdc.gov/mmwr/volumes/67/wr/pdfs/mm6730a3-H.pdf.
Mberu, Blessing U., Tilahun Nigatu Haregu, Catherine Kyobutungi, et al. 2016. "Health and Health-Related Indicators in Slum, Rural, and Urban Communities: A Comparative Analysis." *Global Health Action* 9, 1. https://doi.org/10.3402/gha.v9.33163.
McAlevey, Jane. 2016. *No Shortcuts: Organizing for Power in the New Gilded Age.* Oxford University Press.
McBride, Stephen K., and John M. Shields. 1996. *Dismantling a Nation: The Transition to Corporate Rule in Canada,* 2nd edition. Fernwood Publishing.
McGibbon, Elizabeth (ed.). 2021. *Oppression: A Social Determinant of Health.* Fernwood Publishing.
McGrath, John Michael. 2023. "Ford-Friendly Developers Influenced Greenbelt Changes, Says Auditor General." *TVO Today,* August 9. https://www.tvo.org/article/ford-friendly-developers-influenced-greenbelt-changes-says-auditor-general.
McInnes, Stewart. 1987. *Housing in Canada 1945 to 1986: An Overview and Lessons Learned.* https://publications.gc.ca/collections/collection_2017/schl-cmhc/NH15-518-1987-eng.pdf.
Messing, Karen, and Sylvie de Grosbois. 2001. "Women Workers Confront One-Eyed Science: Building Alliances to Improve Women's Occupational Health." *Women and Health* 33, 1–2. https://doi.org/10.1300/J013v33n01_08.
Migrant Workers Alliance for Change. 2020. *Unheeded Warnings: COVID-19 and Migrant Workers in Canada.* https://migrantworkersalliance.org/wp-content/uploads/2020/06/Unheeded-Warnings-covid19-and-Migrant-Workers.pdf.
Milligan, Kevin, and Tammy Schirle. 2018. "The Evolution of Longevity: Evidence from Canada." *NBER Working Papers* 24929. National Bureau of Economic Research, Inc. https://www.nber.org/papers/w24929.
Mills, C. Wright. 1956. *The Power Elite.* Oxford University Press
Minister of Justice. 2024. *Canada Health Act.* https://laws-lois.justice.gc.ca/PDF/C-6.pdf.
Morrow, Marina H., Olena Hankivsky, and Colleen Varcoe. 2004. "Women and Violence: The Effects of Dismantling the Welfare State." *Critical Social Policy* 24, 3. https://doi.org/10.1177/0261018304044364.

___ (eds.). 2007. *Women's Health in Canada: Critical Perspectives on Theory and Policy*. University of Toronto Press.

Moscrop, David. 2023. "The Greenbelt Report Proves It: The Ford Government Is Corrupt." *TVO Today*, August 9. https://www.tvo.org/article/the-greenbelt-report-proves-it-the-ford-government-is-corrupt.

Mudde, Cas, and Cristóbal Rovira Kaltwasser. 2017. *Populism: A Very Short Introduction*. Oxford University Press.

Muntaner, Carles, and John Lynch. 1999. "Income Inequality, Social Cohesion, and Class Relations: A Critique of Wilkinson's Neo-Durkheimian Research Program." *International Journal of Health Services* 29, 1. https://doi.org/10.2190/G8QW-TT09-67PL-QTNC.

Muntaner, Carles, Orielle Solar, Christophe Vanroelen, et al. 2010. "Unemployment, Informal Work, Precarious Employment, Child Labor, Slavery, and Health Inequalities: Pathways and Mechanisms." *International Journal of Health Services* 40, 2. https://doi.org/10.2190/HS.40.2.h.

Nagpaul, Chaand. 2020. "The Disproportionate Impact of COVID-19 on Ethnic Minority Health care Workers." *BMJ Blogs*. https://blogs.bmj.com/bmj/2020/04/20/chaand-nagpaul-the-disproportionate-impact-of-COVID-19-on-ethnic-minority-health care-workers/.

Navarro, Vicente. 1977. "Social Class, Political Power, and the State and Their Implications in Medicine." *International Journal of Health Services* 7, 2. https://doi.org/10.2190/WPNY-UR3N-0DH9-JTA4.

___. 1986. *Crisis, Health, and Medicine: A Social Critique*. Tavistock Publications Ltd.

___. 2007a. "Neoliberalism as a Class Ideology; Or, the Political Causes of the Growth of Inequalities." *International Journal of Health Services* 37, 1. https://doi.org/10.2190/AP65-X154-4513-R520.

___ (ed.). 2007b. *Neoliberalism, Globalization, and Inequalities: Consequences for Health and Quality of Life*. Baywood Press.

___. 2020. "What Should Be the Objective of an Emancipatory Project?" *International Journal of Health Services* 50, 3: 253–263. https://doi.org/10.1177/0020731420908139.

Navarro, Vicente, Carles Muntaner, Carme Borrell, et al. 2006. "Politics and Health Outcomes." *The Lancet* 368, 9540. https://doi.org/10.1016/S0140-6736(06)69341-0.

Navarro, Vicente, and Leiyu Shi. 2002. "The Political Context of Social Inequalities and Health." In *The Political Economy of Social Inequalities: Consequences for Health and Quality of Life*, edited by Vicente Navarro, 403–418. Baywood.

Naylor, David, Andrew Boozary, and Owen Adams. 2020. "Canadian Federal–Provincial/Territorial Funding of Universal Health Care: Fraught History, Uncertain Future." *Canadian Medical Association Journal* 192, 45. https://www.cmaj.ca/content/cmaj/192/45/E1408.full.pdf.

NCCDH (National Coordinating Centre for Determinants of Health). 2018. *Let's Talk: Racism and Health Equity*, Rev. ed. St. Francis Xavier University. https://nccdh.ca/images/uploads/comments/Lets-Talk-Racism-and-Health-Equity-EN.pdf.

Nelson, Sarah E., and Kathi Wilson. 2017. "The Mental Health of Indigenous Peoples in Canada: A Critical Review of Research." *Social Science and Medicine* 176. https://doi.org/10.1016/j.socscimed.2017.01.021.

OECD (Organisation for Economic Co-operation and Development). 2021. *A New Benchmark for Mental Health Systems: Tackling the Social and Economic Costs of Mental Ill-Health.* OECD Health Policy Studies. Paris: OECD Publishing. https://doi.org/10.1787/4ed890f6-en.

———. 2024a. "Trade Union Density." Data extracted on May 17, 2024, at 16:56 UTC from OECD.Stat. https://stats.oecd.org/Index.aspx?DataSetCode=TUD.

———. 2024b. "Incidence of Low and High Pay." https://doi.org/10.1787/4ead40c7-en. Accessed on May 17, 2024. https://www.oecd.org/en/data/indicators/incidence-of-low-and-high-pay.html.

———. 2024c. "Poverty Rate." https://doi.org/10.1787/7f420b4b-en. Accessed on August 10, 2024. https://www.oecd.org/en/data/indicators/poverty-rate.html?oecdcontrol-8027380c62-var3=2020.

———. 2024d. "Infant Mortality Rates." https://doi.org/10.1787/bd12d298-en. Accessed on May 17, 2024. https://www.oecd.org/en/data/indicators/infant-mortality-rates.html?oecdcontrol-b84ba0ecd2-var3=2020.

Office for National Statistics. n.d. "Coronavirus (COVID-19) Related Deaths by Ethnic Group, England and Wales: 2 March 2020 to 10 April 2020." https://www.ons.gov.uk/peoplepopulationandcommunity/birthsdeathsandmarriages/deaths/articles/coronavirusrelateddeathsbyethnicgroupenglandandwales/2marco20to10april2020.

Office of the Auditor General of Ontario. 2023. *Special Report on Changes to the Greenbelt.* https://www.auditor.on.ca/en/content/specialreports/specialreports/Greenbelt_en.pdf.

OHC (Ontario Health Coalition). 2019. "Briefing note: Doug Ford Government Cuts to Health Care." https://www.ontariohealthcoalition.ca/wp-content/uploads/Briefing-note-on-Fords-cuts-updated-nov-20.pdf.

———. 2023. "Analysis: Ontario Health Coalition Analysis of Bill 60, Your Health Act." Posted March 10, 2023. https://www.ontariohealthcoalition.ca/index.php/analysis-ontario-health-coalition-analysis-of-bill-60-your-health-act/

———. 2024. "Public Hearings on Protecting and Improving Local Hospitals: Community Members Invited to Give Input." June 3. https://www.ontariohealthcoalition.ca/wp-content/uploads/JUN_3_2024_OHC_public_hearings-web-vrsn.pdf.

OHRC (Ontario Human Rights Commission). 2005. *Policy and Guidelines on Racism and Racial Discrimination.* https://www3.ohrc.on.ca/sites/default/files/attachments/Policy_and_guidelines_on_racism_and_racial_discrimination.pdf.

Ontario Federation of Labour. 2023. "Enough Is Enough." https://ofl.ca/enough-is-enough/.

Oved, Marco Chown, Brendan Kennedy, Kenyon Wallace, et al. 2020. "For-Profit Nursing Homes Have Four Times as Many COVID-19 Deaths as City-Run Homes, Star Analysis Finds." *The Star,* May 8.

Oxfam. 2022. *Profiting from Pain: The Urgency of Taxing the Rich Amid a Surge in Billionaire Wealth and a Global Cost-of-Living Crisis.* https://www.oxfam.ca/wp-content/uploads/2022/05/Oxfam-Media-Brief-Profiting-From-Pain-Davos-2022-Part-2.pdf.

Palmer, Bryan. 2023. "Capitalism, Colonialism, Canada: How the Past Is Before Us." *SP The Bullet*. https://socialistproject.ca/2023/01/capitalism-colonialism-canada/.

Panitch, Leo, and Sam Gindin. 2004. "Global Capitalism and American Empire." *Socialist Register* 40.

Paradies, Yin, Jehonathan Ben, Nida Denson, et al. 2015. "Racism as a Determinant of Health: A Systematic Review and Meta-Analysis." *PLoS One* 10, 9. https://doi.org/10.1371/journal.pone.0138511.

Parliament of Canada. 2024. *Bill C-64: An Act Respecting Pharmacare*. House of Commons of Canada. https://www.parl.ca/DocumentViewer/en/44-1/bill/C-64/first-reading.

Peters, Jared (ed.). 2012. *Boom, Bust and Crisis: Labour, Corporate Power and Politics in Canada*. Fernwood Publishing.

Pomeroy, Steve. 2015. *Built to Last: Strengthening the Foundations of Housing in Canada*. Federation of Canadian Municipalities. https://www.homelesshub.ca/resource/built-last-strengthening-foundations-housing-canada.

____. 2021. *Background Primer on Canada's Housing System*. Canadian Housing Evidence Collaborative, Canadian Centre for Housing Rights and Law. https://chec-ccrl.ca/wp-content/uploads/2022/08/Background-Primer-on-Canadas-Housing-system-APRIL-20-2021.pdf.

Poulantzas, Nicos. 2020. "Towards a Democratic Socialism." Translated by Patrick Camiller. *Jacobin*.

Prime Minister of Canada. 2023. "Working Together to Improve Health Care for Canadians." https://www.pm.gc.ca/en/news/news-releases/2023/02/07/working-together-improve-health-care-canadians#:~:text=Canadians%20must%20have%20equitable%20access,%2446.2%20billion%20in%20new%20funding.

Primrose, David, Rodney D. Loeppky, and Robin Chang (eds.). 2024. *The Routledge Handbook of the Political Economy of Health and Health Care*. Taylor and Francis.

Qiu, Theresa, and Grant Schellenberg. 2022. *The Weekly Earnings of Canadian-Born Individuals in Designated Visible Minority and White Categories in the Mid-2010s*. Statistics Canada.

Raphael, Dennis, Toba Bryant, Juha Mikkonen, et al. 2020. *Social Determinants of Health: The Canadian Facts*. Oshawa: Ontario Tech University Faculty of Health Sciences and Toronto: York University School of Health Policy and Management. https://thecanadianfacts.org/The_Canadian_Facts-2nd_ed.pdf.

Raphael, Dennis, and Ambreen Sayani. 2019. "Assuming Policy Responsibility for Health Equity: Local Public Health Action in Ontario, Canada." *Health Promotion International* 34, 2: 215–226. https://doi.org/10.1093/heapro/dax073.

Roh, Jin Soo. 2019. "What Many Canadians Don't Know about the Canada Health Act." *Toronto Star*, January 9.

Scambler, Graham. 2019. "Sociology, Social Class, Health Inequalities, and the Avoidance of 'Classism.'" *Frontiers in Sociology* 4, 56. https://doi.org/10.3389/fsoc.2019.00056.

Scheffler, Richard M., and Daniel R. Arnold. 2019. "Projecting Shortages and Surpluses of Doctors and Nurses in the OECD: What Looms Ahead." *Health Economics, Policy and Law* 14, 2. doi:10.1017/S174413311700055X.

Schimmele, Christoph M., Feng Hou, and Max Stick. 2023. *Poverty among Racialized Groups across Generations*. Statistics Canada.

Schrecker, Ted. 2016. "Neoliberalism and Health: The Linkages and the Dangers." *Sociology Compass* 10, 10. https://doi.org/10.1111/soc4.12408.

Scott-Samuel, Alex, Clare Bambra, Chik Collins, et al. 2014. "The Impact of Thatcherism on Health and Well-Being in Britain." *International Journal of Health Services* 44, 1. https://www.jstor.org/stable/45140692.

Shuttleworth, Joanne. 2023. "Referendum: 98% Against Private, For-Profit Health Care." *Wellington Advertiser*, June 1. https://www.wellingtonadvertiser.com/referendum-98-against-private-for-profit-health care/?utm_source=rssandutm_medium=rssandutm_campaign=referendum-98-against-private-for-profit-health care.

Silverman, Hollie, Konstantin Toropin, Sara Sidner, et al. 2020. "Navajo Nation Surpasses New York State for the Highest COVID-19 Infection Rate in the US." *CNN*, May 18. https://www.cnn.com/2020/05/18/us/navajo-nation-infection-rate-trnd/index.html.

Skilleter, Dan. 2024. *Billionaire Blindspot: How Official Data Understates the Severity of Canadian Wealth Inequality*. Social Capital Partners. April 2024.

Smith, Katherine E. 2007. "Health Inequalities in Scotland and England: The Contrasting Journeys of Ideas from Research into Policy." *Social Science and Medicine* 64, 7. https://doi.org/10.1016/j.socscimed.2006.11.008.

———. 2013a. "Institutional Filters: The Translation and Re-Circulation of Ideas about Health Inequalities within Policy." *Policy and Politics* 41, 1. https://doi.org/10.1332/030557312X655413.

———. 2013b. *Beyond Evidence-Based Policy in Public Health: The Interplay of Ideas*. Springer.

———. 2014. "The Politics of Ideas: The Complex Interplay of Health Inequalities Research and Policy." *Science and Public Policy* 41, 5. https://doi.org/10.1093/scipol/sct085.

Smylie, Janet, and Michelle Firestone. 2016. "The Health of Indigenous Peoples." In *Social Determinants of Health: Canadian Perspectives*, edited by Dennis Raphael, 434–469. Canadian Scholars' Press.

Socialist Project. 2023. "Canadian Workers, the Social-Ecological Crisis and Alternatives." *The Bullet*.

Standing, Guy. 2014. "The Precariat." *Contexts* 13, 4. https://doi.org/10.1177/1536504214558209.

Statistics Canada. 2016. "Unmet Health Care Needs, 2014." February 9. https://www150.statcan.gc.ca/n1/pub/82-625-x/2016001/article/14310-eng.htm.

———. 2018. "Deaths and Causes of Deaths, 2015." *The Daily*, February 23. https://www150.statcan.gc.ca/n1/en/daily-quotidien/180223/dq180223c-eng.pdf?st=hJFtMBbr.

———. 2019a. "Mental Health Care Needs, 2018." https://www150.statcan.gc.ca/n1/en/pub/82-625-x/2019001/article/00011-eng.pdf?st=zZ7HrKFa.

———. 2019b. "Dental Care, 2018." https://www150.statcan.gc.ca/n1/en/pub/82-625-x/2019001/article/00010-eng.pdf?st=4dRlQ3Ep.

———. 2022a. "Home Care Use and Unmet Home Care Needs in Canada, 2021." *The Daily*, August 26. https://www150.statcan.gc.ca/n1/en/daily-quotidien/220826/dq220826a-eng.pdf?st=aENLcdFb.

———. 2022b. "Experiences of Health Care Workers During the COVID-19 Pandemic, September to November 2021." *The Daily*, June 3. https://www150.statcan.gc.ca/n1/en/daily-quotidien/220603/dq220603a-eng.pdf?st=4RicZ5hn.

———. 2022c. "Quality of Employment in Canada: Pay Gap, 1998 to 2021." May 30. https://www150.statcan.gc.ca/n1/en/pub/14-28-0001/2020001/article/00003-eng.pdf?st=mEVXoHub.

———. 2023a. "Canadian Income Survey, 2021. *The Daily*, May 2. https://www150.statcan.gc.ca/n1/en/daily-quotidien/230502/dq230502a-eng.pdf?st=tVxGrOAq.

———. 2023b. "Housing Economic Account, 1961 to 2021." *The Daily*, January 16. https://www150.statcan.gc.ca/n1/en/daily-quotidien/230116/dq230116d-eng.pdf?st=urVi2UfT.

———. 2024a. "Core Housing Need in Canada." https://www150.statcan.gc.ca/n1/pub/11-627-m/11-627-m2022056-eng.htm

———. 2024b. "Distributions of Household Economic Accounts for Income, Consumption, Saving, and Wealth of Canadian Households, First Quarter 2024." *The Daily*, July 17, 2024. https://www150.statcan.gc.ca/n1/daily-quotidien/240717/dq240717a-eng.htm.

———. 2024c. "Labour Force Survey, January 2024." *The Daily*, February 9. https://www150.statcan.gc.ca/n1/en/daily-quotidien/240209/dq240209a-eng.pdf?st=nhXqsMYc.

———. 2024d. "Health of Canadians." https://www150.statcan.gc.ca/n1/en/pub/82-570-x/82-570-x2023001-eng.pdf?st=fFbJUlKB.

———. 2024e. "Unmet Health Care Needs by Sex and Age Group." https://www150.statcan.gc.ca/t1/tbl1/en/tv.action?pid=1310083601.

———. n.d. "National Health Grant Program." https://www66.statcan.gc.ca/eng/1962/196202410223_p.%20223.pdf.

Stephens, Carolyn. 1996. "Healthy Cities or Unhealthy Islands? The Health and Social Implications of Urban Inequality." *Environment and Urbanization* 8, 2. https://doi.org/10.1177/095624789600800211.

Strategic Organizing Center. 2023. *In Denial: Amazon's Continuing Failure to Fix Its Injury Crisis*. https://thesoc.org/what-we-do/in-denial-amazons-continuing-failure-to-fix-its-injury-crisis/

Syed, Iffath Unissa, and Farah Ahmad. 2021. "COVID-19 and Health care Workers' Struggles in Long Term Care Homes." *Journal of Concurrent Disorders* 3, 1. https://cdspress.ca/wp-content/uploads/2021/04/NK09_FINAL.pdf.

Syed, Iffath Unissa, Tamara Daly, Pat Armstrong, et al. 2016. "How Do Work Hierarchies and Strict Divisions of Labour Impact Care Workers' Experiences of Health and Safety? Case Studies of Long-Term Care in Toronto." *Journal of Nursing Home Research* 2, 1. https://www.ncbi.nlm.nih.gov/pmc/articles/PMC5218838/.

Tarasuk, Valerie, Tim Li, and Andrée-Anne Fafard St-Germain. 2022. "Household Food Insecurity in Canada, 2021." Toronto: Research to Identify Policy Options to Reduce Food Insecurity (PROOF). https://proof.utoronto.ca/wp-content/uploads/2022/08/Household-Food-Insecurity-in-Canada-2021-PROOF.pdf.

Tarasuk, Valerie, Andrew Mitchell, Lindsay McLaren, et al. 2013. "Chronic Physical and Mental Health Conditions among Adults May Increase Vulnerability to Household Food Insecurity." *The Journal of Nutrition* 143, 11. https://doi.org/10.3945/jn.113.178483.

Taylor, Dorceta. 2014. *Toxic Communities: Environmental Racism, Industrial Pollution, and Residential Mobility*. New York University Press.

Taylor, Doug. 2011. "The Fight for Medicare in Saskatchewan." YouTube video, May 23. https://www.youtube.com/watch?v=tG9pNoUwtT4.

Thompson, Mitchell. 2023. "Socialism Now Enjoys Widespread Support in Canada, Fraser Institute Says." *PressProgress*. February 23. https://pressprogress.ca/socialism-now-enjoys-widespread-support-in-canada-fraser-institute-says/.

TommyDouglas Tube. 2012. "Saskatchewan Doctors Strike 1962." YouTube video, February 12. https://www.youtube.com/watch?v=D42ZF1mLiGM.

Transnational Institute. 2017. *People Power: 12 Struggles of Resistance and Hope in 2017*. http://2017movements.tni.org.

———. 2018. *People Power: 12 Struggles of Resistance and Hope in 2018*. http://2018movements.tni.org.

U.S. Department of Labor. 2023a. "US Department of Labor Finds Amazon Exposed Workers to Unsafe Conditions, Ergonomic Hazards at Three More Warehouses in Colorado, Idaho, New York." OSHA news release, February 1. https://www.osha.gov/news/newsreleases/national/02012023.

———. 2023b. "U.S. Department of Labor Finds Amazon Failed to Provide Injured Employees Proper Medical Treatment at Castleton, New York, Fulfillment Facility." OSHA news release, April 28. https://www.dol.gov/newsroom/releases/osha/osha20230428.

United Nations. 1999. "UN Human Rights Committee: Concluding Observations: Canada." April 7. CCPR/C/79/Add.105." https://www.refworld.org/docid/3df378764.html.

———. 2007. "United Nations Expert on Adequate Housing Calls for Immediate Attention to Tackle National Housing Crisis in Canada." November 1. https://www.ohchr.org/en/statements/2009/10/united-nations-expert-adequate-housing-calls-immediate-attention-tackle-national.

———. 2016. "Concluding Observations on the 6th Periodic Report of Canada: Committee on Economic, Social and Cultural Rights." https://digitallibrary.un.org/record/831868?ln=en.

Valdes, Francisco. 1996. "Unpacking Hetero-Patriarchy: Tracing the Conflation of Sex, Gender and Sexual Orientation to Its Origins." *Yale Journal of Law and the Humanities* 8, 1. https://core.ac.uk/download/pdf/72833279.pdf.

Veltmeyer, Henry. 2020. "Capitalism, Development, Imperialism, Globalization: A Tale of Four Concepts." *Globalizations* 17, 8. https://doi.org/10.1080/14747731.2019.1699706.

Villermé, Louis-René. [1840] 1988. "A Description of the Physical and Moral State of Workers Employed in Cotton, Wool, and Silk Mills." In *The Challenge of Epidemiology: Issues and Selected Readings*. PAHO/WHO.

Waitzkin, Howard. 2024. "The Transition to Post-Capitalist Health and Health care." In *The Routledge Handbook of the Political Economy of Health and Health care*, edited by David Primrose, Rodney D. Loeppky, and Robin Chang. Taylor and Francis.

Wallace, Maeve, Joia Crear-Perry, Lisa Richardson, et al. 2017. "Separate and Unequal: Structural Racism and Infant Mortality in the US." *Health and Place* 45. https://doi.org/10.1016/j.healthplace.2017.03.012.

Wallace, Rob. 2020. *Dead Epidemiologists: On the Origins of COVID-19*. Monthly Review Press.

Wallace, Rob, Alex Liebman, Luis Fernando Chaves, et al. 2020. "COVID-19 and Circuits of Capital." *Monthly Review*, May 1.

Walt, Gill. 1994. *Health Policy: An Introduction to Process and Power*. Zed Books Ltd.

Whitehead, Margaret, Mark Petticrew, and Hilary Graham. 2004. "Evidence for Public Health Policy on Inequalities: 2: Assembling the Evidence Jigsaw." *Journal of Epidemiology and Community Health* 58, 817–821.

WHO (World Health Organization). 2008. *Closing the Gap in a Generation: Health Equity through Action on the Social Determinants of Health*. https://iris.who.int/bitstream/handle/10665/43943/9789241563703_eng.pdf.

———. 2018. *WHO Housing and Health Guidelines*. https://iris.who.int/bitstream/handle/10665/276001/9789241550376-eng.pdf?sequence=1.

———. 2020. *COVID-19 and Violence Against Women: What the Health Sector/System Can Do*. https://iris.who.int/bitstream/handle/10665/331699/WHO-SRH-20.04-eng.pdf?sequence=1.

———. 2023. *World Health Statistics 2023: Monitoring Health for the SDGS, Sustainable Development Goals*. https://www.who.int/publications/i/item/9789240074323.

———. n.d. "The Global Health Observatory, Life Expectancy at Birth (Years), Metadata" Accessed August 10, 2024. https://www.who.int/data/gho/data/indicators/indicator-details/GHO/life-expectancy-at-birth-(years).

Whyte, Murray. 2020. "'My Parkdale Is Gone': How Gentrification Reached the One Place That Seemed Immune." *The Guardian*, January 14.

Wilkinson, Richard G. 1989. "Class Mortality Differentials, Income Distribution and Trends in Poverty 1921–1981." *Journal of Social Policy* 18, 3. https://doi.org/10.1017/S0047279400017591.

———. 1992. "Income Distribution and Life Expectancy." *BMJ* 304, 6820. https://doi.org/10.1136/bmj.304.6820.165.

———. 1997. "Socioeconomic Determinants of Health: Health Inequalities: Relative or Absolute Material Standards?" *BMJ* 314, 7080. https://doi.org/10.1136/bmj.314.7080.591.

Wilson, Jim. 2023. "Nurses Cite High Stress, Poor Culture, Increasing Workload – Despite End of Pandemic." *Canadian HRReporter*, August 9. https://www.hrreporter.com/focus-areas/compensation-and-benefits/nurses-cite-high-stress-poor-culture-increasing-workload-despite-end-of-pandemic/378603.

Wolff, Richard D., and Stephen A. Resnick. 2012. *Contending Economic Theories: Neoclassical, Keynesian, and Marxian*. MIT Press.

Wood, Ellen Meiksins. 1995. *Capitalism Against Democracy: Renewing Historical Materialism*. Cambridge University Press.

_____. 2017. *The Origin of Capitalism: A Longer View.* Verso.
Wright, Erik Olin. 2015. "How to Be an Anticapitalist Today." *Jacobin.* https://jacobin.com/2015/12/erik-olin-wright-real-utopias-anticapitalism-democracy/.
_____. 2018. *How to Be an Anticapitalist for the 21st Century.* https://www.sscc.wisc.edu/soc/faculty/pages/wright/How%20to%20be%20an%20anticapitalist%20for%20twentiethe%2021st%20century%20--%20full%20draft,%20July%2025%202018.pdf.

Index

academics,
    advocacy struggles, 62, 77, 80, 98, 121
    biases of, 62, 71, 96
    on ideas, 71–2, 77
    policy consultation, 55, 58, 69–71
    privileging opinions of, 59, 62, 73
Alberta, 78, 126
    health care policy in, 34, 36–8
    long-term care in, 45
Albo, Greg, 59–60, 80
Amazon, 85–6
anti-capitalist movements, 114, 117, 134
Arab people, 4, 6, 15, 29
At Home/Chez Soi project, 24, 33n4, 58
austerity measures, government, 39, 47, 89
Australia,
    health policy in, 51, 57–8
    welfare state metrics, 100, 104, 106–7, 109
Austria, 104, 106–7, 109

Belgium, 104, 106–7, 109
Big Capital, 33n3
    activism challenging, 32, 80, 112, 134
    destructive impacts of, 78, 85–6
    neoliberalism and rise of, 20–1, 86
    state/policy support for, 1–2, 50, 54, 64, 86, 119
    workers' movements versus, 80, 86, 112
Bill C-64: An Act Respecting Pharmacare, 43
Black people, 5–6, 15, 79, 88–91
Black Report (UK), 56–7, 70
British Columbia, 77, 91
    health care policy in, 34–5, 37–8, 42–3
    long-term care in, 45
British North America Act, 34
Bryant, Toba, 77

Canada Assistance Plan, 35, 37
Canada Health Act, 39, 131
    critiques of, 42–4, 46
    principles of, 36, 41, 50
Canada Health and Social Transfer, 36–8, 40
Canadian Labour Congress, 23, 36
capital accumulation,
    exploitative drive for, 11, 88–9, 93–5, 98n1, 99n3
    health impacts of, 11, 27, 83–6
    neoliberal housing approaches and, 26–7
    policymaking and, 54, 77, 119
    resistance to, 21, 100, 121
    see also Big Capital; capitalism; capitalist class
capitalism, 79
    class relations under, 15, 31, 33n2, 83–7, 99n3, 119–21
    COVID-19 pandemic and, 97–8
    financialized, 88–90
    health inequities in, 9–10, 49, 82–3, 89–91, 108–10
    ideology of, 3, 18, 21, 50, 77–83, 93, 133–4
    Keynesian economics and, 18–19, 31, 32n1
    liberal-colonial, 87–93
    mercantile, 88
    policymaking under, 21–2, 50, 75–7, 80
    poverty under, 7–10, 12, 108–10
    racism in, *see* racism
    as root of inequities, 1, 62–3, 82–6, 108, 115, 133–4
    sexism and, *see* sexism
    social democracy in, 110–11, 118–19
    socialist activism against, 18, 112–19, 121–6, 133–4

Index 155

state-managed, 18, 75–6, 88–9
struggles against, 75–7, 98, 103, 113–16, 126–8, 132–3
trade unions in, 103–5, 111–12, 130–3
see also anti-capitalist movements; Big Capital; capital accumulation; capitalist class; capitalist states
capitalist class,
better overall health of, 9–10, 84–5
exploitation of workers by, 12, 15, 19, 65, 93–5, 99n3, 121
neoliberalism benefiting, 19–22, 104–5
policymaking influence of, 50–1, 54, 65, 105
profit motives of, 10–11, 83–4, 93–5
state support for, 32, 76–7, 104–5, 110, 119, 134
welfare state approaches to, 101, 103, 110
capitalist states,
ecological and worker harm under, 78, 92–3
health care inequities under, 9–10, 48, 100, 118–20
housing policy under, 25–8, 30–2
Cargill meat plant, 92
Chadwick, Edwin, 9–10, 113
children, 75
harsh living/working conditions, 11, 27, 93
policymaking impacts on, 31, 117
poverty and, 9, 15, 105
racialized/Indigenous, 90, 97
socialism and, 102
Chinese people, 4–6, 15, 89, 92
Christian democratic welfare states, 102–9
civil society groups,
neoliberalization of, 64–5
Clarke, John, 76
class,
awareness, 125, 130
capitalist, see capitalist class
gendered health impacts of, 11–16, 94–5
health impacts of, 9–16, 53, 70, 96–8
housing insecurity and, 28–30
middle, 25, 102

poverty as issue of, 7–8, 15–16
race and health impacts of, 13–16, 60, 96–8
social democratic states and, 100, 111
as social determinant of health, 1, 82, 94–5
struggle, 19, 32, 83, 88, 112–14, 119–20
unequal relations of, 7–13, 70, 83–7, 99n2
welfare state regimes and, 100–2
working, see working class
climate change, 77–8, 126
colonialism,
health impacts of, 13–14, 90–3, 95, 98
inequities due to, 1, 13, 48, 82, 90–3, 96, 133
mobilizing to challenge, 120, 128, 131
practices and evolution of, 87–93, 95
Conservative government (Canada), 24, 58, 78
see also Progressive Conservatives
Conservative government (UK), 57, 118
conservative welfare states, 100–2
with former fascist dictatorships, 103–10
cooperatives, 23, 30, 116
core housing need, 24, 29–30
concept of, 27
see also housing insecurity
corporatism, 54
cost sharing (health care), 35–6, 40
COVID-19 pandemic, 16n3
health inequities and, 7, 10, 50, 91, 95–8
long-term care homes amid, 45, 48, 63–4, 97–8
neoliberal policies and, 47, 94
ongoing impacts of, 25, 28
poverty and, 5, 10, 25, 43, 91–2
racialized community impacts, 13–14, 43, 48, 91–2, 97–8
temporary income support, 5, 40
critical political economy, 1, 59, 99n5, 113
approach to health inequities, 70, 82–3, 98, 119
Crowe, Cathy, 62–3, 66n1

democracies,
    Christian, 102–9
    liberal, 53–4
    policymaking influence in, 53–4, 56
    representative, 52–4, 56
    unions in, 103–4, 111–12, 116
    worker struggles in, 21, 88–9, 122–6, 131–2
democracy,
    ideals of, 52–4, 116, 120, 122, 126
    labour movement/union, 111–12, 124–6, 130–2
democratic socialism, 114–15, 117
Denmark, 100, 104, 106–7, 109
dental care,
    gaps in accessing, 44, 130
    lack of funding for, 42, 44, 46
disabled people, 11, 91, 108, 132
    health/housing supports for, 22, 31, 128
    rights struggles, 55, 126
doctors, 97
    gendered discrimination by, 11
    policy influence and, 57, 61–2, 96
    public health care and, 35–6, 41, 43, 49
    shortage of, 46–8
domestic violence, 11, 95

education, 46, 99n4
    earning gaps and, 5–6, 16n1, 85, 96
    health correlations with, 6, 8, 92, 97, 134
    political/policymaking influence and, 57, 60
    socialist approaches to, 121–2, 134
    unequal distribution of, 4, 31, 97
    worker/public, 111, 113, 118–21, 126, 131
elections, 23–4, 35–8, 43, 118–19
    union, 132
elites,
    neoliberal policies and, 20–1, 35, 80, 134
    policymaking influence, 51, 54, 61–2
    power, 53–4, 76
    socialism versus, 101, 112, 123
Ellwood, Paul, 56
employment, 99n4
    activism for better, 18, 56, 115, 128
    capitalism and, 18–20, 33n2
    factors affecting, 43–4, 77, 92
    full-time versus part-time, 5, 48–9, 85–6, 97, 105–6, 128
    government recommendations on, 56–7
    health care, 48–9, 63–4
    health inequities and, 15, 42, 46, 65, 96–8, 128–9
    housing disparities and, 18–19, 30
    insecure, 10, 12, 14, 47–8, 85–6
    insurance, 92, 128–9
    lack/loss of, 6–7, 10, 16n7, 95
    policymaking and, 18–20, 47, 95, 110, 128
    racial inequities and, 92, 95, 97
    unequal distribution of, 4, 91–2
    unions and, see unions
    wage disparities in, 5, 16n1, 96–7, 105–6
    welfare states and, 101–2
    women's, 5–7, 11–12, 95, 102
Engels, Friedrich, 82, 113–14, 119, 123
epidemiology, 7, 10
Esping-Andersen, Gøsta, 100, 103
evidence,
    influence versus ideology/ideas, 67, 69, 71, 74–81
    policymaking and, 53, 56–9, 65, 75, 84, 134

fascism, see conservative welfare states
Filipino people, 4–7, 15, 79, 96
Finland, 100, 104, 106–9
food insecurity,
    factors in, 15–16, 30
    rates of, 14–15, 129
Ford, Doug, 47
fossil fuel industry, 77–8
France, 44, 100, 104, 106–7, 109, 118
funding, 89
    advocacy biases based on, 62–5, 71
    cuts to, 21, 23–4, 36–41, 47, 64
    health care, 35–7, 36–42, 44–5, 50n1
    for housing, 23–4, 30–2
    privatization and, 35, 41, 47–50

gender, 60, 79, 82
  capitalism's discrimination based on, 1, 12, 32, 53, 97–8, 113–15
  earnings gaps/poverty and, 5–8, 12, 93–4, 96, 99n4
  food/housing insecurity and, 15–16, 28–30
  health inequities and, 8–13, 16n6, 43, 95, 113
  socialism and, 100, 113, 120, 134
  trade unions and, 111, 132
  violence, 11, 94–5
gentrification, 25–6
Germany, 44, 100, 104, 106–7, 108–9
Gindin, Sam, 75, 83–4
Gramsci, Antonio, 119
grassroots movements,
  capitalism versus, 115–16
  policy change and, 59, 65
  socialist, 117, 120, 122
Great Depression, 18–19
Greece, 104, 106–7, 109
Greenbelt scandal, 27

Hall, Peter, 67–9, 72
Hancock, Trevor, 77–8
Harper, Stephen, 24, 38–9
health,
  activism, 121, 123–4
  capitalism impacts on, 9–10, 49, 82–3, 89–91, 108–10
  colonialism impacts on, 13–14, 90–3, 95, 98
  equity, see health equity
  mental, see mental health
  racism impacts on, 8–9, 13–16, 42–3, 89–95, 133–4
  sexism impacts on, 1, 12–13, 82, 93–8, 133
  social determinants of, see social determinants of health
health care,
  costs, 35, 56; see also cost sharing (health care)
  out-of-pocket payment for, 42–3
  perceptions of Canadian, 1, 7, 53, 72, 123
  policies, see health care policies
  private, see private health care
  public, see public health care
  reduced spending on, 36–42, 44–5, 50n1
  universal, see universal health care
  wait times, 38–9, 46, 68
  workers, see workers
health care policies,
  concept of, 52
  four periods of struggle, 50
  influence over, 47, 54
  neoliberalism and, 47, 49–50
  shifts in, 34–8, 40, 47
health coalitions, 36, 61, 64, 127–8
health equity, 85
  approaches to, 50, 52, 117
  mobilizing for, 58–9, 111, 121, 124–5, 126–7
  policymaking and, 50, 55, 71, 74, 80, 123–4
  socialism as path to, 98, 100–3, 113–14, 120, 132–4
health inequities,
  in capitalism, 9–10, 49, 82–3, 89–91, 108–10
  in COVID-19: 7, 10, 50, 91, 95–8
  critical political economy approach to, 70, 82–3, 98, 119
  gender and, 8–13, 16n6, 43, 94–5, 113
  Indigenous, 8, 13–14, 29–31, 91–3, 95
  living conditions and, 1, 9, 12–13, 22, 63, 70, 129
  poverty and, 84–5 108–10, 118, 129
  power and, 4, 16, 63–5, 82, 98, 117–18
  racialization and, 8–9, 13–16, 42–3, 91–3, 133–4
  as socioeconomic and political, 51–2
  worker, 9–10, 15, 42, 46, 65, 96–8, 128–9
health policy, 33n4, 127
  capitalism/neoliberalism impact on, 21, 51, 118
  concept of, 52
  ideas/paradigms and, 67–72, 77, 80
  political power dynamics and, 53–9, 61–5, 74–5, 80–2, 133

health politics, 59, 74, 117, 133
   concept of, 51–2
heteropatriarchy, 16n6, 93, 95
home care, 39, 46, 48–9
homelessness, 90–1
   community mobilizing on, 33n4, 31–2, 63, 76, 129
   government initiative on, 24–5, 32, 63
   policies worsening, 26–7, 58, 63, 68
homeowners,
   housing insecurity, 28–30
   social housing provision and, 23, 25, 31
housing,
   affordable, 22–4, 26–31, 76, 117, 127
   cooperatives, 23, 30
   core need for, *see* core housing need
   insecurity, *see* housing insecurity
   public, 19, 22–6, 30–1, 54, 77
   social, 23–7, 30–2, 58, 65–7, 76, 129, 133
Housing First approach, 24, 62
housing insecurity, 129
   class and, 28, 30
   gender and, 28–9
   government initiative on, 24–5, 31–2, 63
   indigeneity and, 29–30
   persistence of, 28–30, 76, 86
   policies worsening, 26–7, 58, 63, 67–8, 86
   racialization and, 14, 29–30
housing policies, 67–8, 86
   health inequities, 22, 63
   neoliberal, 26, 49, 63
   shifts in Canada's, 22–4, 31–2
Hurley, Michael, 64

ideas,
   concepts of, 71–3
   journeys, policy, 69–72, 128
   neoliberal capitalist, 20–3, 32, 50, 57–8, 76–7, 125
   policymaking and, 38, 42, 53–9, 68–9, 76–81
   reinforcing inequities, 13, 16n6, 32, 74, 91, 132
   research-informed, 59, 67–70, 73–4, 78–9, 133

socialist, 100–2, 110–14, 117–18, 121–3, 130, 133
immigrants, 26, 60
   capitalism impacts on, 33n2, 85, 131
   COVID-19 pandemic, 10, 14, 92, 97
   health care for, 42–3, 97
   status disadvantages, 6, 10, 99n4
   wage/job discrimination, 94–6
imperialism,
   harmful impacts of, 87, 90–1, 133
   struggles against, 93, 120, 131
Indigenous people,
   emancipatory movements of, 126, 131
   health inequities facing, 8, 13–14, 29–31, 91–3, 95
   housing/food insecurity, 15, 29–30
   (neo)colonialism, impacts on, 13–14, 87–93, 98
   policymaking on, 23, 39, 57, 70–1
   poverty rates, 6
   power and representation, lack of, 60–1
inequities,
   economic, 9, 20, 23, 33n2, 88–9
   health, *see* health inequities
infant mortality, 27, 103
   rates, 8, 108–10
insurance, health, 92
   company resistance to public, 34–5
   lack of, 42–4
   privatization of, 47
   public, 41, 74–5
   welfare state regimes and, 100–2
Ireland, 104, 106–9
Italy, 104–9

Japanese people, 1, 4–6

Keynesianism, 18, 32n1
   policy shifts to and from, 19–20, 31, 34–5, 68, 94
Kingdon, John, 55–8
Kirby Committee on health care, 37–8
Korean people, 5–6, 29

Labour Party (UK), 57, 118
Latin American people, 4–6, 14–15

liberal Anglo-Saxon welfare states, 20, 100–2
  poverty/infant mortality in, 108–10
  trade union density/wages in, 103–6
liberal democracies, 20, 53–4
Liberal government (Canada), 24, 35–8, 43
life expectancy, 1, 8–9, 26, 84
living conditions,
  capitalism and inhumane, 27–8, 110
  health inequities and, 1, 9, 12–13, 70, 129
  labour movement organizing and, 126, 128
  socialism and, 110, 123
  see also housing insecurity
lobbying, 53–4, 59, 64
long-term care (LTC) homes,
  advocacy for, 63–4
  in COVID-19 pandemic, 45, 48, 63–4, 97–8
  public versus private ownership of, 44–5
  shortages and working conditions in, 46, 48–9, 96–7
low(er)-income workers, 46, 111
  health/care inequities for, 11, 14–15, 41–4, 92–3, 128–9
  housing problems of, 25–6, 30–1
  pay gaps and, 94, 96, 98
  policymaking and, 22–3, 25–7
  welfare state regimes and, 101

Manitoba, 126, 131
  health care in, 34, 38, 45
  housing in, 23
marginalized groups, 16n7, 99n3
  COVID-19 impacts on, 10, 14
  health inequities for, 14, 38–9, 90–1, 93
  lack of policymaking influence, 60–1, 79
  pay gaps of, 5, 94
  support for, 31, 127
  welfare state regimes and, 89–90
market systems,
  free, 18, 20–1, 63

labour, 5, 33n2, 83–5, 88, 95
  policy influence and, 54, 100, 124
  private, 21, 31, 102
  welfare state regimes and, 100–2
Marx, Karl, 79, 113–14, 119, 123
Marxist economics, 18–19, 119, 123
Medicare, 38, 41
Mehra, Natalie, 60–1, 64
mental health,
  conditions worsening, 13, 43, 83–5, 90–1
  gender and, 11, 94
mental health care,
  gaps in provision of, 13, 43–4, 46
  housing and, 24, 27, 33n4
  policymaking on, 38–9, 58, 129–30
Ministers' Accord on Health Care Renewal, 38–9
Mulroney, Brian, 19, 23, 36–7, 39

National Housing Act (1949): 22
National Housing Strategy (NHS), 24, 33n4, 68
  Act, 25, 32, 131
Navarro, Vincente, 102–3, 113–14
neoclassical economics, 18–19, 35
neoliberalism,
  capitalist class benefiting from, 19–22, 35, 80, 104–5, 134
  COVID-19 and, 47, 94
  health care policies, 21, 47, 49–51, 118
  housing approaches under, 26–7, 49, 63
  ideologies/spheres of, 20–3, 32, 50, 57–8, 76–7, 125
  state support for, 19–20, 39, 134
  wage policies under, 22, 33n2, 65, 83–6, 94–5, 99n3
Netherlands, 100, 104, 106–7, 109
New Brunswick, 37–8, 45, 86
New Democratic Party, 43, 77, 112
Newfoundland, 31, 36, 45, 86, 117–18
Northwest Territories, 37, 45, 48
Norway, 44, 104, 106–7, 109
Nova Scotia, 36, 38, 42, 45
nurses, 12, 96, 123
  labour organizing by, 125–7

policymaking input by, 62–3, 72, 127
privatization and, 48–9
shortage of, 40, 47–8
Nunavut, 1–2, 30–1, 45, 48, 91

oligopolies, 54
Ontario, 60–1, 77
    community mobilizing in, 62–3, 76, 126–8
    COVID-19 impacts in, 14
    health care in, 36, 38, 42–5, 47
    health care worker shortage, 47, 49
    neoliberal/capitalist policymaking in, 27, 47
    union mobilization in, 49, 64, 127–8
Ontario Coalition Against Poverty, 63, 76
Ontario Council of Hospital Unions, 64, 127

Palmer, Bryan, 90
Panitch, Leo, 79, 84
paradigms, 67–72, 77, 80
patriarchy, 1, 11
    hetero, *see* heteropatriarchy
personal support workers (PSWs), 48–9, 62, 97, 123
pharmacare, 37, 42–3
policy,
    academic consultation, 55, 58, 69–72, 77
    capitalist-centric, 1–2, 50–1, 54, 61–4, 86–7, 90, 119
    change in, *see* policy change
    concept of, 52
    evidence-based, 53, 56–9, 65, 75, 84, 134
    health care, *see* health care policies
    health, *see* health policy
    housing, *see* housing policies
    ideologies/ideas and, 67, 69, 73–4, 77–81
    paradigms and, 67–72, 77, 80
    physician consultation, 57, 61–2, 96
    process elements, 67–8
    public versus private, 52
    unequal influence over, 1–2, 50–6, 63–6, 96, 105, 119

policy advocates, 56, 59, 62, 69, 133
policy change, 102
    concept/process of, 51–3, 55–6
    elements of, 67, 76
    health care/housing, 23–4, 35, 37, 43, 59
    incrementalism toward, 52–3, 70–3, 115
    levels of, 67–8, 130–1
    politics and, 52–3, 59, 69, 80
    radical, 36–7, 47, 52, 56–8, 62, 68
    socialist, 113, 123, 128
    streams in process of, 55–8
policy entrepreneurs, 56, 58
policy windows, 56–9
politics, 20, 35
    concepts of, 51–3
    critical political economy approach to, 82, 87, 91
    health, *see* health politics
    impacts on health, 4, 10, 102–3, 111
    participatory, 80, 125–6
    policymaking power and, 52–6, 60, 64, 68–9, 77
    socialist, 118–19
Portugal, 104–7, 109
Poulantzas, Nicos, 119
poverty,
    addressing, 7, 117, 124
    as class issue, 7–9, 15–16, 30, 101, 103
    cycle of, 10
    gendered and racialized, 6, 11–14, 91, 94
    health inequities and, 84–5 108–10, 118, 129
    Indigenous, 6, 90–1
    marginalized experiences of, 25, 27, 51, 57, 94
    policy approaches to, 18–19, 24–5, 85–6, 105–10, 117–18
    rates of, 5–6, 86, 105–8
power,
    colonial state, 87–8, 105
    elite, 53–4, 76
    gendered, 11, 16n6
    health inequities and, 4, 16, 63–5, 82, 98, 117–18

health policy and, 42, 49–55, 63–6,
77–82, 123–4
ideologies/ideas and, 73–4, 77–81
money and, 18, 21, 59–64, 74–5, 78–80,
118
political/economic, 18–22, 47, 69,
74–8, 86–7, 118
socialist redistribution of, 110–13,
116–19, 122, 134
socioeconomic inequities, 33n2,
59–62, 66, 83–4, 115, 133–4
unions' use of, 63, 125–6, 130–2
welfare state dynamics of, 101–3
worker/community struggles for,
19–21, 31, 63–5, 96, 126–7
precariat, 85, 89, 97, 98n1
Prince Edward Island, 37, 42, 45, 86
private health care, 45
insurance, 42–4, 74–6, 101
movement toward, 36–9, 47–50, 76,
133
universal versus, 35, 41, 46, 75, 100
privatization, 7
health care, 36–9, 47–50, 76, 127, 133
housing, 25, 31, 76
neoliberal promotion of, 19–22, 64
wage discrimination and, 94, 99n4
Progressive Conservatives, 23, 36
provinces and territories, Canadian,
federal transfer payments, 36–8, 40
health care in, 34–42, 49, 129–30
movement to public health care, 34–8
public housing in, 22–3, 31
public health care,
doctors in, 35–6, 41, 43, 49
insurance, 34–5, 41, 74–5
neoliberalism and, 47, 49–51
provincial movement to, 34–8

Québec, 30, 45, 60, 126
health care/pharmacare in in, 35–7

race, 100
capitalism's discrimination based on,
1, 12, 32, 53, 97–8, 113–15
earnings differentials and, 5, 16n1,
95–6

health inequities due to, 8–9, 13–16,
42–3, 91–3, 133–4
housing insecurity and, 26, 29–30
poverty and, 6–7, 13–15, 82
union responses to, 111, 132
racialization, process of, 16n7, 88–9
racism, 16n7, 48, 82, 131
health inequities due to, 13, 89–95,
128, 133
systemic, 1, 12–14, 32, 53, 97–8, 113–15
refugees, health care for, 38–9
renters, housing insecurity, 28–30
representation, political, 52, 56, 60, 91,
130–1
resources,
colonial exploitation of, 13, 88
health impacts of lack of, 14, 82, 92
housing and, 26, 119
provincial management of, 36, 40
public policy influence and, 49–52,
60–3, 124
socialist sharing of, 114, 120–2
unequal distribution of, 1, 16n7, 51,
58–62, 76, 110
revolution, societal,
advocacy for, 111–14, 134
class conflict leading to, 18–19, 82, 112
gradual approaches versus, 115–16, 123
Romanow Commission, 37–9
royal commissions on health care/
services, 35, 37
rural communities, 102
health care in, 39, 48
housing in, 23, 28
Russia, 19, 89

Saskatchewan, 34–5, 45
Service Employees International Union
Healthcare, 63, 127
settler colonialism, *see* colonialism
sexism, 16n6
capitalism's discrimination based on,
1, 12–13, 82, 93–8
struggles against, 128, 131, 133
Shelter and Housing Justice Network,
63, 66n1
single-parent families, 6, 15, 26, 28, 46

slums, 27–8
Smith, Katherine, 69–72
social democracy, 110–12, 119
  parties of, 112, 115, 117
social democratic welfare states, 100–2, 105–9
  unions in, 103–4
social determinants of health,
  interconnectedness of, 8, 65
  policymaking and, 51–2, 57–9, 65, 70, 123–4
  unequal distribution of, 4, 52, 57, 59, 82, 134
socialism,
  as alternative to capitalism, 19, 110–16, 118–20, 128
  concept of, 113, 118, 121–3
  democratic, see democratic socialism
  health activism and, 123–5, 130
  health equity and, 19, 98, 103, 114–17, 125, 132–4
  labour movements and, 111–12, 125–6, 130, 133
socialist policies, 128–30, 133
  on medicine, 39–40, 50
  need for, 3, 110, 121
Socialist Project Labour Movement, 3, 130
socialist societies, 120–3, 128
South/East Asian people, 4–6, 15
Spain, 104, 106–9
stagflation, 19–20
state, the, 125
  bottom-up pressure on, 59, 62, 117–18, 122
  capitalist interests and, 27, 49, 64, 76–80, 84, 118–19
  (in)action on health/housing inequities, 31–2, 52, 65, 100, 102
  neoliberalism and, 20, 39, 134
  (non)intervention of, 18–19, 21, 23–4, 32–33nn1,2, 46, 98
  people's struggle against, 112, 114–15, 120
  policymaking considerations, 22, 45, 53–6, 69, 77–8, 134
  responsibilities versus provinces/
territories, see provinces and
  territories, Canadian
Stewart, Sharleen, 63–4, 74, 97
Sweden, 100, 104, 106–7, 109
Switzerland, 104, 106–7, 109

Toronto, 10, 131
  housing issues in, 22, 25–6, 63
Trudeau, Justin, 39
Trudeau, Pierre, 23

unions,
  amid capitalism, 103–5, 111–12, 116, 130–3
  declining membership, 86, 105, 108, 110
  democratic processes in, 111–12, 124–6, 130–2
  mobilization of, 49, 64, 127–8
  societal power dynamics and, 63, 125–6, 130–2
  wage rates and, 86, 89, 103, 105, 108, 110
  welfare state regimes and, 103–6
United Kingdom, 26
  electoral politics in, 57, 118
  unequal policy influence in, 51–3, 56–7, 70, 96
  welfare state metrics, 104, 106–7, 109
United Nations Committee on Economic Social, and Cultural Rights, 24, 32
United States, 75, 88, 118
  health inequities in, 14, 90, 109–10
  health policy change in, 56, 77, 96
  union density, wages, and poverty in, 103–8, 110
  wealth distribution and influence in, 20, 86–7, 90, 100
universal health care,
  fight for, 35, 41, 75
  liberal welfare state limits on, 101–2
  war on, 36–9, 42, 50, 76, 133

wages,
  activism for better, 102, 115, 127–8, 131
  discrimination in, 5, 89, 94
  gaps in, 4–5, 94–5
  housing/food insecurity and, 15

low, 10, 84–6, 95, 105–6, 108
  neoliberal policies and, 22, 33n2, 65, 83–6, 94–5, 99n3
  trade union density and, 86, 89, 103, 105, 108, 110
  women's, 5, 11, 94–5
wealthy people,
  health (care) of, 9–11, 84
  policymaking interests of, 21, 32, 51–4, 76–8, 110
  workers versus, 64, 86–7, 118, 124–5
welfare states,
  Christian democratic, *see* Christian democratic welfare states
  conservative, *see* conservative welfare states
  evolution and dismantling of, 94, 102–3
  liberal, *see* liberal Anglo-Saxon welfare states
  metrics, 103–10
  social democratic, *see* social democratic welfare states
West Asian people, 4, 6, 15, 29
Wilkinson, Richard, 10
women,
  earnings gaps/poverty and, 5–8, 11–14, 91, 93–4, 96, 99n4
  food/housing insecurity and, 15–16, 28–30
  health inequities facing, 11–16, 16n6, 43, 94–5, 113
  medical discrimination facing, 11
  as single parents, 6, 15, 26, 28
  socialism and, 100, 113, 120, 134
  violence against, 11–12, 94–6
  working conditions, 11–12, 111, 132
  see also gender; sexism
workers,
  Big Capital versus, 78, 80, 86, 112
  exploitation of, 12, 15, 19, 65, 92–5, 99n3, 121
  health/care inequities for, 11, 14–15, 41–4, 92–3, 97, 128–9
  lack of policy influence, 61–2
  low(er)-income, *see* low(er)-income workers

migrant, 91–2
organizing of, 21, 88–9, 122–8, 131–2
personal support (PSWs), 48–9, 62, 97, 123
precarious, 85, 89, 97, 98n1
shortage of health care, 47–9
socialism and, 111–13, 118–21, 125–6, 130–3
struggles for power, 19–21, 31, 61–5, 96, 126–7
working class, 102
  health inequities, 9–10, 27, 98
  housing, 25, 27
  neoliberal capitalist policies versus, 20–1, 25, 83–4, 93, 103
  socialist organizing of, 103, 112, 118–19, 130
  solidarity, 7, 125, 130–1
workplaces, 70, 99n4
  capitalist, 7, 11, 13, 45, 110, 131
  harmful conditions in, 11–12, 47–9, 75, 96, 127
  injuries in, 9, 11, 85–6
  mobilizing workers in, 80, 49, 92, 112, 115, 124, 128–31
  sexism in, 11–12, 94
  see also employment
World War I: 19, 34
World War II, 19, 87
  health/housing policy after, 34, 20, 22–3
Wright, Erik Olin, 114–15

Yukon, 45, 48